Nine Years After

Jeff Block

DEDICATED TO DEBBIE

These are the words and opinions of the author who stands behind
everything he has said

CHAPTER 1

The mornings are the absolute worst. Waiting. I may appear comfortable as I sit at my computer console. A cup of coffee is well within reach, so are some cookies. The news of the world slowly scrolls by on the screen speaking of murders, terrorist atrocities, wars, political strategies and intrigues and the latest Hollywood gossip. I absorb it all without making a sound. If I had my way the stereo would be playing and sweet music would waft through the house and overshadow this silence of waiting. Yet the silence is integral to the waiting. Without the silence I would be unable to hear the snores of Debbie asleep in what used to be our bedroom. Sometimes I still stand by the bedroom door to ensure that what I am hearing is Debbie's continued breathing. It is. I release a deep sigh and wander back to the computer in the kitchen. The keyboard strokes silently as the minutes of the morning slip away.

I am usually fully awake by seven. There is a stack of library books by the futon that I have accepted as my bedroom. I read voraciously. Tons of fiction from around the world mixed with real life biographies. The stories remind me of the pain and heartbreak that encompass the daily lives of my fellow human beings. For brief moments I find an escape from my own overpowering depression. An hour or so of reading in the morning while I snuggle within the warmth of my blankets and overlying quilts. I remain quiet. Quiet enough so that I can distinguish the sounds from my beloved Debbie's breathing. The sounds are harsh actually, a deep nasal snore that awakens me several times each night as I try to sleep through on my futon which lies a few feet from the bedroom door. It seems like years since I have had an uninterrupted night's sleep. It has been years.

In addition, these days I am awakened by our aged cat C.C. who has made it her habit to climb atop my face and to continue returning despite my efforts at getting her to refrain from this obnoxious habit. Invariably I arise and pour some milk into her bowl. This buys me another half hour or so of blessed sleep before the whole cat dance begins again. Eventually enough half hours of sleep accumulate to equal the five or six hours I have become accustomed to. I arise and brew the coffee that will kick start my day into gear. The first sip is in me by eight.

I read and acknowledge the events of the world. Nothing much new this morning. The conservatives are still harping about the cost of health care. Must be nice to be a congressman and be able to depend on the government for your family's health care.

Shame they can't see their way clear to allowing the rest of us to have the same benefit. Anyway, the key thing for me is to remain silent. Debbie's requirements for sleep are not the same as mine and I must not disturb her rest. Nine A.M. has become ten and ten has become eleven. Eleven creeps closer to noon and I begin to expect to hear the sliding of Debbie's booties as she makes her way out of the bedroom. I am ready for her. I, as always, have made sure that there will be a fresh cup of coffee for her. Some days this means I have had to brew a second pot having drunk the first one by myself. Some days eleven A.M. slips right past noon without Debbie's appearance. Panic usually strikes me by 11:30 forcing me to once again ensure that Debbie still breathes. My body shivers with dread as I listen at the bedroom door. Yes, Debbie is still breathing today.

I consider waking her but I am wary. I have learned from experience that it is to my benefit to allow Debbie to awake at her own speed. Grouchy is a weak way to describe Debbie if she hasn't obtained her desired 12-15 hours of sleep a day. I know that if I awaken her prematurely the rest of her waking hours will be full of recriminations for the chores I have left untended any time in the fourteen years plus of our marriage. I am amazed that Debbie can remember, let alone care, that on our first St. Patrick's Day as a wedded couple that I prepared corned beef for dinner. Didn't I know that she hates corned beef? Believe me when I say that I know it now. And God forbid that I ever mention the word liver. I remember once saying the word river. Debbie misunderstood and thought I said liver. Her protest was long, angry and venomous. I've never made the mistake of cooking liver for her and I haven't had any myself for years now. Giving up liver has not been a difficult sacrifice for me. Remaining silent has. Silence is still the name of the game as the daylight hours pass. I remain alert to every sound.

Today the outdoors is as quiet as indoors. Heavy fog has invaded the valley in which we live. An occasional droplet of moisture falls from the eaves of our Blue Ridge Mountain home. I can't even see across the valley to our neighbors. The fog has muffled and silenced even the birds. No sound disturbs Debbie's continuing sleep that has now extended into the thirteenth hour. I check on her once more. Her snoring continues. I wonder how she can sleep through that racket she makes. She swears she doesn't snore. She didn't use to, but she sure does now. My silence continues as does my morning and now early afternoon vigil.

Some days the silence is smashed by the ring of the telephone. I am quick enough to pick up before the third ring. My heart actually jumps at the prospect of speaking with someone. Maybe the tedium of the days will be broken with the excitement of seeing a friend. Invariably, however, I am disappointed by the recorded messages of bill collectors or fundraisers. I gently hang the phone back in its cradle checking to be sure that the phone's intrusion has not awakened Debbie. She sleeps still.

Some days the silence is broken by a boom. Debbie has fallen again. I am at her side within seconds. She is bruised again but otherwise unhurt. I can read the history of her falls in the colors of her body. The deep purples are the recent falls, the light blues that meld with browns and yellow are the older ones that have almost healed. Often the colors of the bruises shade into each other making the old marks indistinguishable from the newer ones. After all, there really are but so many ways in which a body can crumple to the ground. Percentages say that usually you land on your ass. Debbie's ass, which has given me such pleasure through the years, is now a colorful work worthy of the country's best kindergarten finger painters. Debbie's confusion at her predicament is tangible. I can feel her wondering, once again, how did I end up here? I relax her, make sure there is nothing hurt or broken and once convinced that there is nothing but another bruise to further color the canvas that was once her unmarked body, I help her to stand again using the two hands crossed in an "X" method that we have perfected. I count three and lift as Debbie wobbles her still unsteady legs into an upright position.

Most days thankfully do not begin with a booming fall. Most days begin with several hours of silence as I wait for Debbie to awaken. Most days begin with me sipping coffee at the computer and waiting. I know in my heart that these days cannot continue forever. I know that one morning Debbie will not be breathing. I dread that day. I pray for the postponement of that day. I know that fulfillment of that prayer just extends the long parade of depressing and sleepless nights followed by days that are more than half spent by the time I can break my silence. I pray for the patience that will allow me to endure this day. I pray for the compassion required to curb my anger at this continuing abomination of silence. I pray for a future I no longer believe in.

Debbie is a brain cancer patient and has been for the last nine years and for me, it is the mornings that are the absolute worst.

CHAPTER 2

Deborah Sylvia Clark was born in Syracuse, New York on February 26, 1955. She is nearly a full year younger than I who was born on March 12, 1954. The president of the United States was Dwight Eisenhower and Jonas Salk was in the field of disease prevention. Salk invented and perfected a vaccine for polio that allowed both Debbie and I the opportunity to play outdoors with other children as we grew up- a fact of which we were both blissfully unaware at the time. The year I was born was the same year that Willie Mays roamed centerfield for the New York baseball Giants and made his famous over the shoulder catch to spark the Giants to a World Series championship. Debbie's birth year witnessed at least two miracles- her birth and the ascendancy of the Brooklyn Dodgers to their first and only baseball championship. I was born and raised in Brooklyn. The Dodgers left in 1958. I stayed until 1977.

Debbie's time in Syracuse is mostly forgotten. She is the fourth of five children born to Donald and Virginia Clark. Donald was an insurance man and work kept him hopping from place to place as the family grew around him. Virginia juggled the demands of her five children with a full time nursing job.

The most vivid memory Debbie has of these days in upstate New York were of a large meadow that was their backyard. She speaks fondly of times playing in the snow. Certainly there were sibling rivalries with which Virginia would have had to stop her housework and play referee. Older brothers Dean and Brad would have been incorrigible and the teasing of Jennifer, Debbie and Robin must have been incessant. None of this was abnormal though. The few photographs that have survived this era show the Clarks gathered at birthdays and Christmases with presents and wrappings galore and with smiling children. Pictures show the older children taking turns holding baby Robin in their protective grasps.

My first few years were spent in a high-rise apartment building in the Coney Island section of Brooklyn. I am the second of four children. I am guessing that my older brother Lenny and I shared a room in that apartment but I really don't recall. I remember the elevator that we rode up to our floor and I remember a fenced in balcony that we shared with the other inhabitants of our floor. You could see the ocean from there. I remember enjoying the view and must have spent some time playing with other toddlers out there. My mother tells of how one day I came into the house reciting the Hail Mary that I must have been taught by one of my toddler playmates. This was an abomination in our Jewish household and my mother claims that it was the major impetus behind our family's move from Coney Island to the Canarsie section of Brooklyn. I think it more likely that the real reason we moved was a need for greater space after the birth of my twin sisters Roberta and Audrey in 1958.

I do not recollect any idea I had of my mother's pregnancy. I just remember that one day she left the house and returned a few days later with two baby girls. I would grow up, attend school and Hebrew school, achieve my bar mitzvah and graduate from Canarsie High School. My parents continued to live there after I left for the Blue Ridge in 1977 and remained until my father's retirement at which time they migrated to South Florida.

Debbie's father Don was an ardent gardener. He spent many an hour tilling, planting, weeding, pruning and mulching. He tried to interest Debbie in this passion. It did not take for Debbie at the time, which is a great irony, as gardening and landscaping not only became Debbie's profession but it also is her passion.

Perhaps there was a schism of sorts between Debbie and her parents at the time. There have been hints that there was some fighting and tension within the family but if that is so, I feel that that it was not out of the ordinary. For certain, there was a heck of a lot more yelling going on at my house than in hers. I remember one time when I was in junior high and I called my mom to tell her I was at a friend's home around the corner. Her high pitched scream startled me so badly I dropped the phone and all my friends and I could hear her even though we had walked to the opposite end of the room. All families have fireworks and all children rebel against their parents in some way. I truly don't think either Debbie or I were unique in our upraising.

Debbie's father's work forced the Clarks to do some jumping around. The family spent some time in Hartford, Connecticut before transferring south where they were stationed for a piece outside of Atlanta before moving on to Charlotte, North Carolina. Debbie never really speaks of her childhood. The moving around must have been disconcerting on some level but she appears none the worse for it. Eventually Debbie's family came to settle in Cary, North Carolina, a suburb of the state capital, Raleigh. It is here where Debbie went to and graduated from Cary High School and it is here she first fell in love and married.

My father, George, was an auto mechanic and despite the wishes of his parents, opened up a garage instead of becoming a rabbi as his older brother had. The gas station was his haven. It was his place where he was the boss and there were no arguments about that. He hired others who became his most loyal followers and admirers. There was a Puerto Rican fellow, a Black guy, a Mexican, a Chinese at one time, an Italian teenager and his girlfriend who became one of the first female auto mechanics in New York City and even had a write up in the newspaper. It was a regular United Nations down there and I was thrust right into it by the age of six. It was my job back then to go with my father to the station on Sundays. I would pump gas and hustle for tips by cleaning driver's windshields with a squeegee. I bet I was real cute!

Work at my father's station was a constant for me until I left New York. My responsibilities and hours grew as I aged. By the time I was driving I was managing the station when my father would take weekends off and driving the AAA tow truck providing emergency service to stranded motorists.

One Sunday morning I showed up late for work and my father reamed me out a new asshole. I tried to explain that I had gotten in home late the night before from a date with Elyse who became my first wife. Dad didn't want to hear a bit of it. His only concern was my responsibility to the work. He didn't care what, who or how much of anything I did as long as I showed up for work on time and ready. I was never late again and I had learned a great lesson about the differences between lifestyle and life. As long as I put in my hours efficiently and competently I was a man and the rest of my time was my own. What a beautiful concept! It is one I wish would be embraced by my neighbors and countrymen today.

Debbie and I each found our ways into a first marriage that did not last. There are some children who grow up knowing just exactly what they wish too be when they grow up. My brother Lenny was like that. He wanted to be a doctor and he became one. Some couples know that they will remain together forever when they are first introduced in the second grade. Debbie and I, and I think a large majority of us, have absolutely no clue as to our eventual occupations and have no idea as to how to make love last.

Both Debbie and I were cuckolded. Our respective spouses found others to excite their lusts. Bob, Debbie's first husband, at least had the courtesy to marry his paramour. My first wife, Elyse, just slept around. The final straw for me came when I discovered she had slept with a mutual friend of ours. Obviously, Elyse and I were not working out and when she told me she wished to return north I did not stand in her way. In fact, I helped her pack and assisted her in carrying her luggage to her car. I watched as she drove out of my life and felt nothing but relief. The only lasting good that came from my first marriage is that it brought me to the Blue Ridge, which I have considered home ever since. Thank you, Elyse, for taking your graduate degree in the mountains of North Carolina. And thank you, Bob, for leaving Debbie. It may have taken years but we'd have never gotten together had either of us remained married.

CHAPTER 3

Debbie and I have never quite been able to determine the exact day that we met. We have narrowed it down to a two or three year range sometime in the early eighties. Although I think it may be exactly 1981, Debbie is not so sure of that and she has convinced me that I'm not so sure either. We do agree on the city of our meeting. That would be Raleigh, North Carolina. We also agree that we met at a party being held on Raymond Street. Now, I'm pretty sure I had no idea where this place was, or who most of the people were. For that matter I'm pretty sure that I didn't know any of the people there. The party did have a unifying theme. Almost all the people there were planning to travel to Hampton, Virginia the next morning to see the Grateful Dead perform in concert. This was my plan too. I was traveling with my friend Mike who had lived in Raleigh before his wanderings introduced him to the Blue Ridge. Sometime during that evening I'm sure that Debbie and I were introduced. We both agree that we remember none of that and that we had made absolutely no impact upon each other whatsoever.

Now, don't you know, that Debbie has told me that from that very moment she thought I was hot. I am pretty sure that this is revisionist on her part. Sometimes, despite her usual commandeering way, something sweet slips out and I am touched by the innocent syrupy and childlike way that Debbie can on occasion cut through the haze that surrounds her emotions and make a statement that once again reveals her heart and fills my life with meaning. Most times, of course, our communications are limited to her requests for something to make her more comfortable.

Anyway, that first meeting was uneventful other than as a bookmark for us later. Our relationship did not take off in leaps and bounds. We were not blinded by the bliss of love at first sight. If we spoke at all that first evening the words vanished into the ether as quickly as they were uttered. If the smell of Debbie's hair lingered in my mind I was unaware of its origin or even of its presence. If I had said something witty then Debbie made no acknowledgment of it. I have wished that I could remember more of that night. After all, it was the night that I met my wife and the love of my life. It was just a gathering of folks who shared a common interest in music and in revolutionary and off the grid lifestyles. I had a good time.

The next few weeks found me on the concert tour. I spent many nights seeing the Dead perform. I would usually take a month off from my shop in the spring to travel with the minstrels, gypsies, hippies, jugglers, storytellers and clowns who would follow the endless caravan of the concert tour. I'd find time for some summer, fall and wintertime shows also, but the spring tour for me was my nod to the spirit of growth and reawakening from winter doldrums. Anywhere from twenty to thirty days away from work, responsibility or any concern of the world other than myself. Fifteen to twenty nights of concerts enveloped in the communal vibrations of belonging. Admittedly, people who follow a rock and roll band are not your average nine to fivers. Yet, at the shows and in the parking lots, campgrounds and hotels at which these people gathered there was a sense of family. There were no strangers among those who followed. We were all friends and you did not need worry if you had consumed too much of whatever. Your friends, whether you knew them or not, would take care of you just as you would help a fellow traveler who needed assistance. I have never felt so free as I did during those times of the extended road trip. You may rest assured that the memory of the blonde haired girl named Debbie I had met in Raleigh before the Hampton shows had been forgotten by the time the tour reached Philadelphia, New York, Hartford or Maine. Did Debbie dwell on the brown haired handsome man named Jeff she had met? I sincerely doubt that.

And it's there that the whole story might end except for one thing. "Who are the Grateful Dead and why are they following me around?" was a popular bumper sticker for the heads back in the day. Yes, the Grateful Dead, like Christmas and the Fourth of July were a fixture on the calendar. Spring follows winter, Dead tour starts up again and I was once more on the road for my yearly journey through the concert venues of the northeast. Hampton, Virginia for reasons explainable to none became a starting point for many of the Dead's tours in the 80's. Raleigh being on the way to Hampton and also being the home of many of the Carolina's part time heads became a stopping point for me many years running. And so, Debbie and I met again every April. Somehow or other we became aware of each other. I still wish I could conjure up the remembrance of that magic. I can't.

I remember a large party of several hundred held at some farm near to Raleigh. There was a house and a barn. A makeshift stage had been erected and a group of musicians were playing to the crowd that had gathered. By this time I knew a fair amount of the folks. Many of them had Blue Ridge connections too. I also know that Debbie was at this party. We probably acknowledged each other sometime that night but that was it. We just had no spark between us and we each went our separate way.

I do remember the first moment I realized that Debbie was different than the others. It happened the year a group of us rented a beach suite for the Hampton run. I am convinced this was 1984. It was wonderfully fun and relaxing to come from the intensity of the show to the tranquility of the surf. One afternoon between shows Debbie and I walked alone together down the beach. After a short walk, we lied down together on the warm sand, and promptly fell asleep in each other's arms. We had yet to kiss or truly touch, but we had slept together. I woke refreshed and happy. It is a feeling I have very seldom these days.

Somehow however in 1986 things heated up a bit. Maybe it was the stars, maybe it was just the familiarity we had achieved two or three meetings a year for five or six years, but once again I was on my way to start another spring tour in Hampton and Debbie was also planning to go to the shows. I had already obtained a hotel room reservation and

Debbie had not. I asked her if she would wish to share a room with me for the Hampton layover. She agreed.

We went to the show together that evening. We danced together as the familiar tunes we had come to love played through the night. We joined in the communal roar when the band resurrected an older tune that had not been heard in several years worth of shows. We smiled, we laughed, we held hands. We left the Coliseum in a euphoric state of joy. Debbie was wearing a pair of sneakers with a picture of Supergirl upon them. They would squeak as she walked. We held each other by the waist and giggled as Debbie stomped through the puddles of rain soaking both of our blue jeans thoroughly. I began to call her my Supergirl by the time we had reached the perimeter of the parking lot. We walked on the few blocks to our hotel room and it may be the most magical quarter mile of my life. As soon as we had reached our room our wet and soaked pants came off in a rush. Needless to say and not to dwell on the obvious, but, after that night I always knew who Debbie was. She was my Supergirl.

And that should be that, but no! We still lived 200 miles apart, had jobs, sometimes had other relationships going, and nothing came of that brilliant incandescence of a tour weekend in Virginia. It took ten more years for Debbie to agree to marry me.

CHAPTER 4

Today will be a breakout day. We are getting outdoors. It is a few days past Christmas and the New Year of 2011 is just around the corner. The snow that fell delightfully on Christmas morning has remained, until this morning, plastered in white pillowy mounds. Debbie has not even stepped foot on the front porch let alone attempted the icy stairs that lead down to the drifted snow. She has continued her regimen of fourteen hours of sleep, three or four hours of television watching, a two-hour nap, dinner, a rental movie and then bed again. I am going to force her out the door today. I am going to disturb her routine. I am going to make her get up from the bed. I am going to endure her complaints of being too tired. I am going to stand over her and insist that she take a shower. It will be her first one in over a week. I will help her step safely into the bathtub and will stand watch just outside the bathroom door as the shower runs. I will be there when the shower faucet is turned off and I will help her get out of the shower. We will use the hands crossed in an "X" pattern that helps me support her weight while she wobbily steps out of the tub. I will marvel aloud at the wonders of her nude body and exclaim at the contours of her derriere. I will touch her. She will look at me as a child. Somewhere back in her lost memories she recognizes that our touching used to lead us into hours of pleasant lovemaking. We both know now that there will be none of that. I will shed another silent tear as the pain of my enforced celibacy fogs my mind with sadness.

Debbie is completely oblivious to the passage of time. She does not recognize that it does take her nearly ninety minutes to get dressed and ready to leave the house. I will endure her complaints that she could have slept an hour longer knowing that if she had we would be late for the three o'clock physical therapy appointment that we have scheduled for her and that has already been postponed three times this week because of our snowy driveway. I will remind her to continue moving forward with her dressing process. I will remind her again and again to continue getting dressed. I will dissuade her as she first places on her lounging around pajamas and I will remind her once again of her appointment. I will listen as she explains painstakingly that she first wishes to sit and watch TV and have a cup of coffee before she dresses. Once more I will urge her to get dressed to go and then she can have coffee and breakfast. Twenty more minutes will pass as Debbie removes her pajamas that had taken twenty minutes to get on in the first place. I will beg, cajole and wheedle every action from her.

I will watch as she takes her daily medications. I will bite my tongue as she meticulously moves her pills from their pharmacy bottles into a compartmentalized pillbox. I will not even bother to ask her why she just can't take the pills without this added step. I will endure the torture of just wasting another ten to fifteen minutes while she does it.

Of course, I know why she does it. Several years back her mother suggested this to Debbie as a method to help her control her medication schedule. I opposed this action immediately for two reasons. First of all, I am from the don't fix what ain't broke school. Debbie hadn't been missing any medications so I wondered then as I wonder now as to why we should screw up a good routine. Secondly, I was opposed to the extra step of moving pills from one place to another for no apparent reason. The problem of misidentification of pills was and remains my concern. I also was concerned that the extra handling would lead to droppage and spills of her prescriptions. Many are the mornings where I have searched for pills that have fallen onto the carpet or rolled under the bed. Forgive me, what I meant to say is many are the late mornings and early afternoons in which I have had to search for lost pills. Each time I got up from my knees and then had to compare the newly found pill with its companions to be totally certain and sure that Debbie was not doubling up on medications. I would ask her once again why she had to indulge in this extra bit of insanity. She would say that it helps her. I would ask plaintively how does my finding lost pills help her and she would just state adamantly that it does help her. She would agree that I was right in my concern that she would lose or mistake her pills, agree that the old method used to work well, tell me again that I was right. Of course, the next morning, or that is, one o' clock in the afternoon for the rest of us, she would repeat the process of moving the pills once more and meticulously count out a single pill from each prescription bottle and move them to her plastic compartmentalized pillbox. Why can't she just take out a pill and put it in her mouth? It is a mystery. Perhaps she does it because she knows that it drives me crazy to watch her do it.

I am going to repeat at least twenty times in the next hour that her physical therapy appointments are hers and that it is her responsibility to be on time. I will remind her that she does not have time to watch television this morning and I will urge her to continue placing on the four or five layers of clothing she thinks she will need in order to negotiate the fifteen feet between our doorstep and our car which I will have driven back up to the top of our rapidly melting drive. I wait as patiently as I can manage while Debbie removes her three outer layers so that she may return one last time to the toilet. Another ten minutes will pass and Debbie will reemerge from the back bathroom. She will then turn right back and sit back upon the commode to squeeze out the last few drops. Another ten minutes will pass and I will get Debbie in the car. I expect we will be right on time for our three o'clock appointment. She will go to the bathroom again once she arrives at the physical therapy center ensuring that her hour-long therapy session will now only last forty-five minutes.

Debbie's routine does include weekly physical therapy appointments. She has been working with the same therapist for several years now and Katherine is well aware of Debbie's limitations and can accurately gage whether or not Debbie has been maintaining the regimen of home strengthening exercises with which she has been entrusted.   Katherine will not be surprised at Debbie's weakness this afternoon. Katherine and I both know that Debbie's home exercises consist of lifting the remote control to change the channel. The winter and snow have been taking their toll upon Debbie's reserves. Debbie, of course, is oblivious to the weakness her continued inactivity has created.

I am glad for the therapy sessions. It does create a sense of purpose for Debbie and she does become embarrassed at her inability to duplicate exercises she had been able to accomplish in the past. She will swear to Katherine, and to me, that she will work harder in the upcoming week to do her home exercises and that she will not fight with me when I ask that she do them. I almost wish we could just skip this reaffirmation of will. I already know that the Debbie who resides in the shell of a bruised body that almost resembles my wife is not going to do a thing.

Still I am going to take advantage of this break in the below freezing temperatures and force Debbie to move. After all, the forty-five minutes Debbie will be with Katherine will allow me to get the grocery shopping done. The week of enforced imprisonment due to the snowfall has left us low on milk. And besides, the few moments I steal as I walk up and down the grocery aisles are the only moments of independence that I will have this week. I maintain the fantasy that some kind woman will notice me searching the produce and offer to hear my life story over dinner. I long to talk with someone. Anyone.

Most of the cashiers recognize me and know of Debbie's illness and my care taking of her. They ask me of Debbie's progress. I answer politely and appreciate their concern but I do wish that just once someone would ask me how I feel- and mean it!

Yes, it is another day in paradise. I can see the brown ground materializing in patches as last week's snow melts away. The silence is broken by nothing but the sound of our furnace blowing hot air. Noon approaches and I will awaken Debbie for this giant expedition out of our front door and to her therapy appointment. A new calendar will be gracing the work space above my computer console in just two more days and I ask myself once more as I have been asking now for years- does the excitement ever start?

CHAPTER 5

Today is 1/1/11 or as it is sometimes said, one, one, one-one. Last night was New Year's Eve. A typical, yet totally atypical day for yesterday Debbie showed me one of those flashes of creativity and sweetness that made me fall in love with her in the first place. She made me cry.

The day began as it usually does. Silently. Debbie did not awake until nearly half past twelve in the afternoon. An unexpected thaw had brought the temperature to just above fifty degrees and I was determined that we take advantage of the suddenly melted driveway to get outdoors and to make a circle of the walking path at our nearby park. We both know that it is my consistent insistence that Debbie walk as much as possible that has allowed her the ability to walk at all. I announced my intention to Debbie the same moment I handed her a cup of coffee. She acknowledged my plea and stated she would get ready as quickly as she could.

The next two hours saw Debbie complete the turkey sandwich I had prepared for her breakfast and reheating her original cup of coffee five different times in the microwave and returning with the newly warmed brew to her easy chair in front of the television screen. As the hour approached three I reiterated my request that we get outdoors. Debbie finally and grudgingly began to put shoes on her feet.

The park was idyllic. The unexpected warmth had brought forth many others who had been snowbound just a few days before. There were still patches of snow lying in the pasture that in warmer times served the community as a soccer field. Debbie reached for my hand for greater balance as she negotiated the slushy remainders of the last snowstorm of the previous year. We enjoyed watching the dog whose family tormented it by casually throwing the stick it had so eagerly retrieved from the half frozen river. The dog seemed to not mind the cold water and practiced belly flopping across floating ice floes. It was warm enough that we sat and lingered several times on the benches that allow Debbie the opportunity to regain her strength and to stop the trembling in weakened legs before announcing that she is ready to walk again.

We returned home and I started up the stereo. I did this quickly upon our arrival. I needed to have some music this day. I had to have the soul cleansing that my complete immersion into the music allows. I knew that I'd be singing along to the stereo letting my emotions dictate the sound of my voice. It is a way for me to deal with the repressed feelings of sadness and depression that have become me. I went directly to the stereo while Debbie was still sitting by the front door and unlacing her shoes. I hurried because I knew if I let Debbie get to her easy chair then she would have grabbed the remote and flipped on the television and my opportunity for musical release would be gone.

I had chosen to listen to a copy of a New Years concert from many years ago by the Grateful Dead. I expected that the vibe from that long ago New Year would be compatible for my wishes for the coming new year. I have become emotionally worn down as these days of care taking have scraped my senses raw. I can't hide the pain I feel anymore. It is an ever-present component of who and what I have become. I have tried to mask the pain, yet it seeks an outlet. I let it free with the music, attempting to harmonize and become one with the larger sphere of consciousness which surrounds us all. The tears that always linger in waiting found their way down my cheeks as I sang aloud in what I knew was truly my prayer for inspiration when faced with mysteries so misunderstood, dark and vast. My prayer had been uttered with complete honesty. I had sung it out loud with all my heart and was washed by the tears of my sincerity.

And at that moment when all my defenses were down and I had allowed myself to be stripped to my emotional core, that is when Debbie said she had something to give me. Now, I knew that she had been working on a handmade New Year's card for me. She asked for supplies a few days before and I allowed her the privacy to work alone. I wanted her "surprise" to be as surprising as it could possibly have a chance to be.

The handmade greeting card has been something Debbie has always been fond of. She made one for my birthday, for Valentine's Day, our wedding anniversary, for Christmas and Hanukkah and sometimes for just no apparent reason whatsoever. I have always cherished them and our house is decorated with old cards that I have hung and placed on any available flat surfaces that will hold them. In the last few years the cards have become more and more reminiscent of the scribblings of pre-kindergarten children. Debbie's coordination no longer allows her to write legibly and though her effort is apparent the results are childlike.

On our honeymoon, Debbie and I had a remarkable trip through the western states. We chose to stay on in Yellowstone National Park where we were enchanted by the fabulous landscapes, soothed in natural hot springs, awed by the geysers and stunned by the multitude of wildlife. We were privileged to have seen bears of both the grizzly and brown varieties, buffalo, herds of deer, porcupines, foxes, and elk by the dozens. For reasons unexplainable to us both, however, we were taken in by our sightings of moose. I coined a song on the spot and repeated it endlessly to our giggling amusement. "My baby saw a moose, my baby gets a goose!" We would sing our little jingle and then caress each other's behinds enjoying our song and our gooses. By the end of our stay we had seen four moose in their natural environment and our song became "my baby saw four mooses, my baby gets four gooses!" Four times the fun and four times the goosing led to caressing that led to sweet lovemaking. Incredibly enough, our song has endured and Debbie will still respond "Yeah" to complete the couplet.

I opened up the makeshift envelope that Debbie had meticulously created from a piece of paper and scotch tape carefully unwrapping it from her handiwork inside. Her latest card was a blue piece of construction paper folded in quarters. She had found a characterized picture of a moose that she had glued painstakingly on the first page of her card. Underneath in her nearly illegible lettering I could make out the words- Happy Moose Year! Inside I could read the words I Love You! Totally recognizing the effort these scrawls had entailed I burst into a fresh wellspring of tears and affection. Her punning of moose year with New Year had caught me off guard reminding me of the delightfulness of Debbie's humor which has been eroded by the ravages of her illness. We held each other tight for several long moments until Debbie's unsteadiness forced her to let go and regain her seat upon her easy chair. She had reminded me why I continue to endure the dreariness of my days. I do it for her.

CHAPTER 6

The spring of 1995 found me planning once more to join the caravan of travelers again and to see the Grateful Dead. They were going to perform a three-day run of shows in Charlotte, North Carolina only a two-hour drive from my home in the mountains. Naturally I thought of Debbie as I had for the last fifteen years or so when the band came through our neck of the woods. We had been road companions almost yearly now for at least a decade. We had shared many good times and had withstood some bad ones too. One year Debbie's car broke down on the way to meeting me for concerts in Washington, D.C. She called for help and I drove down I-95 to retrieve her and on the way to pick her up, my car broke down too. Somehow, we managed to get both cars back to Washington and weren't even late for the show.

Debbie agreed to join me in Charlotte and although I told her that many of my friends from Boone would be joining us, Debbie was excited to be part of the party. I arranged hotel rooms for the crowd we would be arriving with.

Debbie and I placed our stuff in one of the allotted rooms, our friends squeezed into the other two rooms. Something had changed and I recognized that I approved. In the past, we would have shared the room with others as a way to cut expenses and in recognition of our communal joining. Debbie indicated to me that she wished for us to stay alone.

We all rode together to the first night's show and sat together. After the concert ended we all rode back together and the group of us gathered in the room adjacent to ours where we had a cold beer or two and decompressed from the excitement of the concert. After awhile Debbie said she was ready for bed and asked me to take her. At that moment it became clear to all that the long friendship that Debbie and I had was now moving into a newer phase. One of our friends asked if he and his wife could crash in our room and Debbie said no. Later that year I thanked that couple profusely for their understanding in not making a scene when Debbie expressed her desire for me so plainly and publicly. I told them that their kindness paved the way for our eventual marriage.

Debbie led me away and into bed. Our lovemaking that night had a tenderness that had eluded us in the past. Somehow we both recognized that this wasn't just casual sex anymore. We held each other tight the night through and when we emerged to join the others for breakfast the next morning we had a glow that was visible to our friends. We accepted a fair amount of good-natured teasing and we did not mind.

The three-day run passed in a blur. Debbie and I had clearly stepped from being sometime friends to becoming a lifelong couple. It was a magical stretch. The most important part came when we were preparing to leave to return home. Debbie accepted my request that I come visit her at her home outside Raleigh in a few weeks. Neither one of us had said anything about maintaining and continuing our relationship in the past. It had always just been taken for granted that we would see each other "next time" and that we would continue as we had. This time was different. We both understood we had started something special and new and that we were obligated to discover exactly where this rare and different relationship would lead us.

I began commuting to Raleigh almost every weekend. In the next several months Debbie and I spent more time together than we had in the previous fifteen years. We cooked meals together, we enjoyed restaurants, we danced at local clubs, we stayed up late talking endlessly and we made love with a reckless abandon we had both been unaware we could create together. We took endless pleasure in pleasing and satisfying one another. Our caresses were intended to excite, titillate and tease to stupefying climaxes- and they did.

Debbie's house was located next to a railroad track. The trains were required by law to blow their horns to alert motorists at the railroad crossing at the corner of Debbie's block. We would listen for the train and try to guess whether it was a passenger or a freight train. The one who guessed correctly was entitled to choose whether to please the other or to be pleasured by the other. Being competitive, we both wanted to be the one who guessed correctly. Having become lovers as well as friends the winner always chose to pleasure the other. Several trains a day came by Debbie's house. I had never been able to sustain such prolonged loving before. We were insatiable. We did it in every room of Debbie's house, sometimes rolling off the sofa or bed we had started on, but continuing non-stop after our fall to the floor.

The days spent back at home alone were intolerable. Debbie had accepted my love- finally! I could not wait for the weekends to arrive so that I could leave work and return to Debbie's arms. One time my car blew a tire on the high speed run down the interstate and I was a few hours late. Debbie welcomed me in a way I could have only dreamed of in the past. I wanted to be with her all the time yet somehow I knew to bide my time and wait for Debbie to make the next move.

As Christmas and winter vacation neared I expected Debbie and I to spend the week together. Debbie told me she had arranged to spend the holiday with her mother in Florida. I stood still and speechless for a moment and then Debbie asked me if I would wish to travel with her.

Our trip began from Raleigh and we began to thread our way through South Carolina. We stopped for lunch in a town named Florence and I began to ask Debbie questions about her family. I wanted to know how best to impress her mother. Debbie told me not to worry as she intended to tell her mom and the rest of her family that it was her intention to move in with me that spring. This was a wonderful surprise for me. I had not expected our relationship to move quite as quickly as it had, but I was thrilled. I asked if this meant we were engaged and Debbie in her sensible manner said no, this would be an experiment. I agreed and continued to remain calm but inside my chest my heart was soaring.

My meeting with my mother-in-law to be (I hoped) went very well. Virginia had just purchased a hot tub and had welcomed us with the news that she had preheated the water and encouraged the two of us to soak together as soon as we had eaten. On Christmas day presents were exchanged and even I was the recipient of some small trinkets. Debbie's mom was friendly and welcoming and accepted the news of our living together with happiness.

Winter passed. Debbie had given notice to her employers and although they were disappointed to lose her skills they were pleased that Debbie had found love. When it came time for Debbie to leave they awarded her with a plaque commemorating her years of service and a travel voucher that Debbie and I used to take a four-day cruise to the Bahamas.

Debbie and I spent many hours discussing our best option. Would it be better for her to join me in the mountains or for me to join her in Raleigh? I was willing to do anything and told Debbie I was ready to move. Debbie told me nothing doing. She had always wanted to live in the mountains and she was coming west to join me in the Blue Ridge. She moved at the beginning of June. The experiment she had spoken of at first just never had a chance. Debbie had already agreed to marry me during one of her spring visits up the mountain. We were sitting at a bench and sharing an ice cream in the Blowing Rock town park when Debbie announced we were now engaged and could begin planning not only her move up the mountain, but could begin making the arrangements for our wedding.

Our wedding was held on the last day of August 1996. We had secured the rental of a bed and breakfast just a few miles from our house and had planned an outdoor ceremony to be held. We fretted daily throughout the summer as we endured rain every day in July and August. Miraculously the rains stopped on the 29th and our wedding went off without a hitch. It was not only a successful joining of Debbie and I but was also a reunion for our respective families.

I remember my mother and sisters tapping their feet rhythmically and in unison as they listened to a song by the Grateful Dead. My mother had given me hell over the years for spending so much time seeing those guys, this was the first time she had ever heard them and it turned out she liked the music. I enjoyed informing her just exactly who it was she was tapping her foot to.

Every now and then a loud burst of laughter would erupt and each time I looked over I saw my father in the center of the group that had convulsed out loud. I wandered over and saw my father going to each of our guests and asking if he might share his baby picture with them. They would politely agree to look and he would take out his wallet and carefully remove a brown and faded photo of a baby. The group would "ooh" appreciatively and then my father would move his thumb revealing a baby with a huge penis. It was this that caused the outbursts of joyous howling.

The children of our friends mingled with our young nephews and nieces and played about on the grassy slope while their parents all shared in the happiness that Debbie and I felt. We had created a small universe that day where the sun always shone, the music never stopped, the beer kegs flowed and everyone was awash in love and joy.

Debbie and I left on our honeymoon the next morning. We camped our way across the country after a first night's stay in Chicago where we took in a White Sox game, had dinner on the pier and racked up the largest bar tab of my life in a blues bar that we helped close down near dawn. We made stops in the Black Hills of South Dakota, the Badlands, Mt. Rushmore and Devil's Tower in Wyoming. Each night we lay joyfully and shared one of the bottles of champagne that had survived the wedding party. We continued into the Grand Tetons and Yellowstone where we saw the four mooses we still sing about today. We spent a night in the lodge at Old Faithful and heard complaints from our neighbors that our lovemaking was too loud. We quieted but we didn't stop. We continued into Idaho and spent a day wandering the volcanic caves of the Craters of the Moon. Time was calling us back to our responsibilities back home so we finished our journey with a day trip to Bryce Canyon in Utah and finished our western swing with a stop at the Grand Canyon. The last evening before we began traveling east and home found us standing alone in a deserted section of the rim of the Grand Canyon with a rainbow stretching across the canyon, a full moon rising above it, and miles of orange and yellow clouds extending above and behind us. Holding Debbie and being a part of this incredible natural display may very well be the quintessential moment of my entire life.

I have often wondered just what it was that had changed in Charlotte a year before our wedding. I don't think I will ever know. The story of Debbie and I is the story of how acquaintanceship becomes friendship and friendship becomes love and devotion. What caused that quantum leap? I don't and will never know. I do know that it is a good thing Debbie and I made it when we did. It was probably our last chance. Jerry Garcia, the lead guitarist and acknowledged leader of the Grateful Dead, died in the summer of 1995 and although the other band members continued to play on, the Grateful Dead never toured again. There would be no "next time". Debbie and I had found our love with not a show or a second to spare.

CHAPTER 7

Happiness is nothing but the positive acceptance of one's environment and Debbie and I were happy with our lives as we began them anew as a married couple. We were both working. Debbie had acquired a position as a crew landscaper and I was content in my social work position. We had schedules that usually allowed us to spend our evenings and weekends together, our dual sources of income were more than enough to cover the expenses of our home and we were healthy.

Debbie enjoyed her move to the Blue Ridge Mountains. She immediately began work on new flowerbeds around our home to brighten the landscape and she joined me in the long walks through the many trails that thread their way through the forests and across the ridge tops. We spent many weekends exhausting ourselves as we made our way from vista to waterfalls to mountain meadow. We would find a beautiful spot along some trail and then we would ensure our privacy by bushwhacking our way further uphill so that we could make believe that we were the only two people in the entire universe. We would spread out the snacks and sandwiches I carried in a knapsack on my back and enjoy long hours of just being alone with each other and the peaceful and beautiful surroundings. Debbie would have me carry both a bird and a flower guide and she made a concerted effort to learn the names of the wild mountain flowers she had been unaware of. If it was warm enough we would undress each other and cuddle and caress our way through the hot afternoon. We would return to civilization with the sunset and after enjoying dinners made with our own hands we would fall asleep contentedly wrapped in each other's bodies.

We started a small garden in our front yard. We did not have much space but we were able to grow some lettuce, basil and other herbs. We tried tomatoes almost yearly, but even when they did grow, the rabbits ate them long before we ever did. Debbie, amazingly, would work all day in flowerbeds and still manage to spend a half hour or so a day weeding out our small patch of produce.

Debbie had me purchase some birdfeeders that we spaced around our house. We have spent hours over the years watching the birds flitting and fighting with one another for our gifts of seeds. Debbie spent hours over the guidebooks identifying the various species that found their way to our yard. We both loved the brilliance of the cardinals and laughed at their skittishness whenever any other bird approached. The cardinals would fly away if even the tiniest sparrow came near. We came to recognize the tufted head of the titmouse, the black and gray of the chickadee, the orange belly of the towhee and the pigeon like appearance of the mourning dove. Some days we were treated to the brilliant blue of an indigo bunting or the unexpected yellow of a goldfinch and occasionally a hawk would cruise by searching for lunch. We also set hummingbird feeders in the warmer months and enjoyed their antics as they zipped and swooped and buzzed right over our heads.

One of our wedding gifts had been a bread making machine and Debbie put it to good use. We worked together measuring out the flour and yeast for inclusion in the mix. We loved the smell as the bread began to bake and were thrilled with the flavor of our homemade breads. We tried many different varieties and Debbie became quite a baker.

Both Debbie and I had a fondness for cold beer on hot days, Debbie more than I. She would cap a brew almost as soon as she walked back in the door after her long days on the job. On an average night she would finish five or six bottles on her own while I would sip on one or two an evening. After awhile I began to realize that the cost of our drinking was becoming prohibitive and I searched for alternative ways to maintain our habit. I discovered the joys of home brewing. We purchased the rather small amount of equipment necessary and attempted our first batch of home brewed beer. We were thrilled! The beer we made was excellent and for the next several years Debbie and I never purchased grocery store beer again. We made over three hundred batches of beer, about a batch per week. Each batch produced nearly fifty bottles of beer or just a tinge over two cases worth. We took pride in our innovative beer recipes and created styles for the seasons. Our standard of excellence was a brown ale, but we were making porters, stouts, lights and darks, and special beers for the seasons. We gathered blackberries for a light fruity brew, and one winter gathered fresh spruce for a Christmas beer. We did an oregano beer that was perfect with spaghetti and lasagnas. Our pumpkin spice beer was fabulously refreshing on summer days. We tried many different recipes over the years and were never disappointed. Friends came by and marveled at how well our little kitchen brewery was producing.

There were some evenings during summer seasons when our garden provided the lettuce for our salads, our bread had been hand made and flavored the way we desired and our beer was brewed through our own efforts. I was aware of how unique this was in our pre-packaged and processed American society and the awareness of our happiness would cause me to smile and to turn my head so that Debbie would not witness the tears of joy that came unbidden to my eyes.

Debbie was promoted after just one season working on a crew. She became the boss of a horticultural crew and began to practice some Spanish phrases so that she could communicate more effectively with her migrant crew workers. Debbie was meticulous in her ways and stubborn enough that she made sure things were done to her satisfaction. If it was good enough for Debbie, it was good enough for anyone and Debbie's employers were more than satisfied with her efforts. She received a small pay raise each and every year that she worked and was given an additional Christmas bonus yearly.

Debbie's work schedule also allowed two months off every winter. We began taking winter vacations to sunnier climates. We visited Florida and Debbie's mother every Christmas and one year had the opportunity to see New Orleans where we caught beads at a Mardi Gras parade. We had such a great time there. I remember that one night as we walked from Bourbon Street to the riverfront we stopped to embrace at a street corner. A car pulled alongside the curb and a passenger yelled at us that we should get a room. We laughed our heads off. To think, that amid all the hoopla of the New Orleans French Quarter a few days before Fat Tuesday, it was a middle aged couple-Debbie and I- who were stretching the boundaries of acceptable public displays of affection!

I still did not have the same luck with my jobs as Debbie seemed to. It was a couple or three years after our marriage that I was laid off from my social worker position. Debbie was completely understanding and because we had always lived frugally and well within our income this lay off did not create any real economic hardship. We had paid off Debbie's outstanding credit card balance the first year of our marriage.

It was accepted that I would continue to seek interviews until I was working again. It was frustrating to me to have been placed once again on the job market when I had been doing so well in providing care and guidance to the children who had been entrusted to my care. Several of the children-clients continued to call for me several years after I was dismissed and no longer had any sanctioned influence in their lives. They just trusted me more than any other when they needed advice and counsel. Some weeks I would spend several hours talking on the phone with children in distress and encouraging them to maintain standards and seek the help they still were entitled to by law. I did not resent this time, in fact I was honored, but I did rue that I could not bill the agency for my time.

I found another job soon enough working as an assistant store manager for a nationwide health and vitamin chain. I was an instant success and although I was not as happy in my work as I had been I did not mind the endless stream of customers who wandered in and gave me some people to talk with throughout the days. I missed the outdoor adventure activities I had engaged in with the children but I still loved the outdoor adventures that I engaged in with Debbie.

Occasionally we would take extended weekends when our schedules allowed us to do so. We would arrange accommodations and travel short distances to see concerts or to try our hiking skills on different trails. We cavorted with the deer at the Big Meadows of Shenandoah but were equally at home in the blues bars of Memphis. Debbie had also enjoyed her first ever baseball game we saw together in Chicago and we made several trips over the years to root in person for the Atlanta Braves or the New York Mets. Debbie also enjoyed a visit to Yankee Stadium where she was entertained more by the antics of the fans in our section than she was in the game. The fans would begin a rhythmic clapping and cheer every time the beer vendor made an appearance near our aisle- "Al-co-ho-lics, clap, clap, clap, clap, clap!" Debbie still isn't able to explain why the outfielders should try to throw to a "cut-off" man (to prevent the batter-runner from advancing an extra base) but she did learn to recognize the nine positions and she did seem to understand a force play. We developed a liking for a band named "moe." and arranged some of our weekend trips in order to see them perform. We had become a married couple but we still had our rock and roll roots.

Many of our trips away involved our visiting our families. Since they were spread out along the east coast from Florida to New Hampshire we had many opportunities to make stops along the way to satisfy our cravings for some urban type excitement to help balance out the peaceful and quiet times we had at home. We were always glad to see our friends and family as we traveled about but overall we much preferred our mountain haven and were glad that Debbie had decided to move up to join me rather than the opposite.

Saturday mornings were delicious. Debbie would not have to wake early for work and she would drowse alongside me into the later hours of the morning. She would awaken and would take comfort in the nearness of my body and she would make love to me in a fashion as sweet as maple syrup.

The days passed quickly enough and the hours I spent wandering the mountainsides with Debbie alongside me were delightful. We had occasional spats about things neither one of us could remember now if our lives depended on that remembrance, but we always made up quickly. We never went to sleep angry at one another and we always slept together cuddling and entwined. We were happy.

CHAPTER 8

Debbie and I celebrated our fifth wedding anniversary on the last day of August 2001. It had been my desire, as it always is, to grace the occasion with something a little out of the ordinary. It was the first year that Debbie and I had been computer active and I used the Internet to help me research a place we could stay that would be serene, attractive, private and romantic. I had the idea that we should take a small getaway and I arranged for the rental of a vacation cabin in the Southern Appalachians. The cabin was situated on a large piece of acreage that we would have free rein to hike and cavort upon. It came equipped with a full kitchen and all necessary cooking and serving utensils. It had a front porch with a rocking chaise and a peaceful view of green meadows with the beginnings of fall flowers like ironweed that stood purple among the yellow sunflowers. There was an outdoor hot tub with Jacuzzi attachments large enough for both of us to lie fully under the hot soothing water.

I had purchased enough groceries to keep us eating well for at least two weeks. There were enough cases of beer and bottles of wine to keep us in an alcoholic stupor for a month. Everything was packed into our trunk and Debbie had no clue as to our getaway until the morning of our anniversary when I asked her to gather her luggage for a weekend retreat. She seemed a bit bewildered at first, she had just assumed that we would just go to a local restaurant for dinner, but soon joined in the spirit of adventure and we were on our way. Her surprise was complete.

I had been worried that Debbie would not like the cabin I had finally decided upon. It was rustic, not fancy, but it did have a certain charm. I talked up the idea of a private escape from phone calls and commercialism during the two-hour drive from our home. I spoke of how I wished to be with her, just her, and to have absolutely no interruptions from our enjoyment of each other. I spoke of my continuing desire for her and of how much I craved the deliciousness of her kisses and the never ending and continuous need I had to lay beside her and to lose myself in the lusciousness of her body. I reminded her of how she was my Supergirl and that I had never been satisfied by anyone in the way she satisfied me. My words must have had some impact. Debbie was enchanted with our accommodations and our destination.

Upon arriving we unpacked the groceries and our suitcases and enjoyed a short walk, hand in hand, through and across the grassy fields that adjoined the cabin. We had a beer together and I prepared lunch for us as we waited for the hot tub to heat up to our desired level of temperature. We were comfortable with our surroundings and with ourselves. Sharing another beer we finished our sandwiches and Debbie suggested our first hot tub of the weekend. I followed her like a puppy as she went to the bedroom and stripped off her blue jeans and blouse. Her soft blonde hair fell down to her shoulders. I admired her body and went to hug her nakedness next to mine. The electricity I had felt from her for years still conducted itself directly to my brain and to my nether regions. We slipped into the hot tub, my desire for my beautiful wife clearly apparent.

We soaked for several hours. Occasionally I would leave the tub and return with some snacks and a fresh bottle of our homebrewed beer. We watched the sunset from the tub. Debbie would alternately lie in the water and then sit upon the edge of the tub to cool herself off. Her nipples would stiffen in the cooler air and I would gently suck them into my mouth licking the chlorinated water from them. She would settle back down then into the hot water the white froth of the foaming jets reheating her body and giving me the chance to cool off and slow my jets. We repeated the process several times until we became hungry. Debbie remained in the tub while I slipped on a pair of shorts and began to grille us some steaks.

We ate dinner on the front porch of our hideaway, watching the stars appear one by one. The night air was filled with the sound of crickets and absolutely nothing else except the beating of our hearts. We had managed to survive the first five years of our marriage intact. We had not broken up nor had we divorced. We had not been led astray by others. Our love for each other remained as it had been. Complete and totally satisfactory. Neither one of us would have changed a thing at that moment. We were still in love with each other and with our lives together.

Inevitably our desire led us indoors and our shorts and t-shirts lie in a jagged line between the front porch and the bed. We made love and all was right with our world. We satisfied ourselves several times during that long night and fell asleep finally with Debbie spooned into me, my arm wrapped across her breast, the perfume of our love enveloping us and her hair tickling my nose as I nuzzled her neck. We were content. We slept.

By the next evening our lives had changed forever. Things would never be the same and I would never make love to a woman with a full head of hair again.

CHAPTER 9

The next morning I awoke before Debbie and set a fresh pot of coffee to begin dripping. Debbie joined me not long after the coffee was ready. We sat peacefully enjoying the swinging chaise together and feeling comfortable with our togetherness. I made us breakfast and we ate while planning a short excursion to the nearest village to have lunch. I elected to jump back into the hot tub for a quick soaking and Debbie said she would be just fine continuing to sip at her coffee and orange juice while swinging in the chaise.

I had not been in the water longer than five minutes when I was distracted by a banging sound repeating itself in an arrhythmic pattern. It was almost as if clothes in a dryer were bouncing around and their buttons were banging the interior of the barrel. I had taken my glasses off before entering the water so when I glanced toward the chaise all I could make out was Debbie's shape. I called out to her. She did not respond. I grabbed my eyeglasses and could see Debbie's head banging back against the chaise. That was the cause of the strange noise I had heard. I jumped dripping from the tub and ran to her. Her eyes were rolled back up into her head. Her head was continuing to bang itself against the headrest of the chaise. I seized her shoulders and gave her a quick shake. There was no response. I stood shocked and stunned for a few precious seconds before I realized that Debbie was in the midst of a grand mal seizure. She had, fortunately it turns out, wedged her legs beneath her and it was this that prevented her from being thrown to the ground by the violence of her seizing. Having ensured myself that Debbie's perch was secure and that there was nothing my voice or touch could do to snap her out of her unconsciousness I placed a pillow behind her head to cushion the blows she was continuing to administer to herself and then rushed inside the cabin to use the telephone to dial 911.

The operator asked me to describe the emergency and I explained how my wife had just begun an unexpected and inexplicable grand mal seizure. The operator had me repeat the directions to the rental cabin and I recited the exact directions that had allowed me to drive right up to it. The operator assured me that help was on the way. I went back to the front porch and held Debbie as best I could without trying to move her from the locked in position that was fortuitously protecting her from a fall to the ground. I called her name. The tears were pouring down my face as I held her. Her body jerked uncontrollably. I held her, repeated her name and cried. Debbie had never before had any type of epileptic or seizure experience. Something was terribly wrong and I have never felt as useless and inadequate as I did in those moments of waiting for the ambulance to arrive. In fact, where the hell where those guys?

At least twenty minutes had passed, Debbie was still seizing in violent jerks, her eyes completely white. I left her when I heard the phone ringing. It was the 911 operator inquiring if we still needed medical assistance. "Yes," I responded with all the urgency and vehemence that this situation required. The operator explained to me that many of their calls become false alarms as the patient spontaneously awakens from their distress. She specifically asked if drugs had been involved. "No!" was my emphatic reply. The operator then said she would dispatch the ambulance immediately and I flew into a rage. I could not believe the callousness of these people who were entrusted with providing emergency care. My strong and previously healthy wife was disintegrating into a quivering mass of flesh before my eyes and these people were cold heartedly considering whether it would be worth their while to save her. My feelings of inadequacy, of not being able to help when my help was needed the most intensified. I continued to hold Debbie so that at the very least some portion of her mind would inform her that she was not alone.

Fifteen minutes more and we were still alone when the phone rang once more. This time it was the ambulance driver requesting directions. He kept asking me about the names of various roads and streets with which I was totally unfamiliar. I lost it completely. I reiterated the directions that had allowed me, a stranger to their county, to drive directly to the correct location and I insisted that they do the same thing. The driver then asked me the same questions about drugs. I respected the need for the ambulance technicians to be as fully aware of the situation they were about to be presented with as possible, yet I was disturbed that they had not yet arrived to actually deal with that situation.

Finally I saw the ambulance beginning the climb up the driveway to the front porch of the cabin. They saw Debbie and asked how long the seizure had been going on. I explained that it had been an hour since I called and that Debbie had been unconscious and seizing the entire time. We once again did the drug inquiry dance. "No, my wife doesn't do drugs, now help her damn it!"

I admit that once the medical technicians began to work, they worked quickly and efficiently. They placed Debbie onto their stretcher and carried her into the back of the ambulance. They told me where they were going and insisted that I follow behind them. I refused and told them I was staying with Debbie and riding with her. They could tell I meant it and compromised by saying that I could not ride in the back of the ambulance as my presence would cramp their working space but that I could ride up front with the driver.

One of the emergency technicians climbed aboard with Debbie and had begun to prepare an injection even before the driver had negotiated the k-turn that allowed him to drive down the way he had come. The needle, the first of hundreds to come, was placed in Debbie's thigh. Almost instantaneously, her eyes rolled back to their normal position and her jerking about came to an abrupt conclusion. The driver explained to me that Debbie had been injected with a shot of liquid librium that is used to curtail seizures. It sure did work! The technician asked Debbie if she could hear him. She could. I asked

Debbie if she could hear me. She could. I explained she was in an ambulance on her way to the hospital. She seemed to understand. Debbie, of course, has no recollection of this ride or of any of the events of the next three days.

The ride to the nearest hospital was a short one. The two emergency technicians wheeled Debbie directly into the emergency room where several nurses began attending her immediately. I never saw or heard from those two ambulance men again. Although I was grateful for their expertise and their competence once they realized the gravity of the situation I still find it difficult to forgive them the delay in their arrival. What if Debbie had been the victim of a drug overdose or reaction? Would her life then not have been worth saving? What if her heartbeat had seized up along with the rest of her body? She'd have died while awaiting the ambulance's arrival.

The reaction of the nursing staff was totally different. They had Debbie wired up to several different machines within minutes. They informed me that as soon as they had stabilized Debbie's condition she would undergo a CAT scan. They allowed me to stay by Debbie's side. Debbie was now coherent and recognized my presence. The nurses explained the CAT procedure to us. Debbie acknowledged that it was appropriate for her condition. She remains unaware of this.

Debbie was wheeled into the CAT scan. One of the nurses gave me a chicken salad sandwich to eat as she explained that we were in for a long day. She recognized that I was bordering on shock and she stood by me while I ate asking questions about our life. Her name, if ever I was aware of it, has been lost but her kindness will never be forgotten. This paragon of human kindness asked if I could deal with the necessary paperwork while Debbie was undergoing her scan.

I went to an office where someone asked for our essential information. Name, address, insurance information. I explained that we did have health insurance that had been issued by Debbie's employer but that because of the urgency and confusion of our appearance at the hospital I had not gathered my wallet and therefore could not currently provide the needed insurance information. The woman marked down that we had no insurance. This was not the truth, but the absence of the insurance card at the time of Debbie's initial presentation may have had a factor in Debbie's subsequent care. Whether for better or worse we will discuss further a bit later in the narrative.

In any case the efficiency of the hospital staff continued. Within minutes of Debbie's return from the CAT scan a doctor appeared with a copy of the picture taken of Debbie's brain. He explained to both Debbie and I that a tumor of approximately 3-4 inches had grown inside her brain and had inevitably reached a size that caused it to interfere with the brain's normal activities. It was this tumor that had caused the seizure. He had already informed the nearest regional hospital that was equipped for brain surgery. He told us that we would be immediately ambulanced to Mission St. Joe hospital in Asheville and that a neurosurgeon would meet us in the emergency room. Debbie remembers neither the discussion nor the ride.

For the second time that day we rode together in an ambulance. Debbie in the stretcher in the back and me in the front seat turned toward the back and trying to maintain a conversation with Debbie. She did not seem worried or scared. It was clear that something had taken place and that she knew that. She just hadn't been able to process it yet.

The doctor met us upon our arrival in Asheville. He introduced himself as a neurosurgeon and he already had a copy of Debbie's CAT scan in hand. He showed us the picture of the tumor and told us we had two options. I asked what those options were and he said that we could operate on the brain and remove the tumor tomorrow or we could operate on the brain and remove the tumor next week. He was quite matter of fact and unemotional in his speech. I asked what the benefits of waiting a week would be and he explained that some people wished to have that time to get their affairs in order. He explained that Debbie could be maintained for that week if we desired to do that. I asked if it wouldn't be better to do the operation sooner than later and he agreed that would probably be the best course of action. He said the operation, which was called a craniotomy, would be scheduled for early the next morning and would probably take up most of the day. He explained the procedure that involved drilling a hole through Debbie's skull, removing a portion of her skull that would be reattached upon the operations' conclusion, and the cutting out of the invasive tumor. He explained that there were extremely severe ramifications of this surgery. Debbie could lose her memory, her ability to walk, hear, see, feel, smell or talk. She could become a bedridden vegetable. She could die. He explained, however, that if we left the tumor intact, that is if we did not choose to have Debbie undergo the operation, then the tumor's growth would continue unabated and that Debbie's life expectancy at that point would be no more than several months. Having no real choice, we agreed to the operation and I signed the necessary release forms. Debbie did consent verbally to the operation, but she has no recollection of the conversation or its ramifications.

Debbie was taken away to the NICU or Neurological Intensive Care Unit. I was told that I would not be allowed to stay there with Debbie and several nurses and security personnel made sure that I was escorted from the ward that had been designated as the NICU. They explained that Debbie would be watched carefully and allowed to sleep in preparation for her upcoming brain surgery. My last view of her that evening was of her body attached to various machines all blinking, squeaking and buzzing with the information of her vitals. Various cables and electrical leads shrouded her face so that I could not see it. I told her I'd see her in the morning. She didn't respond.

I was now alone. I was a hundred miles from home, forty miles from my car. I had no identification and I had no money. All that had been left back at the cabin in the hastiness of our departure. Fortunately, Debbie and I had many friends in the Asheville area and I was able to prevail upon the kindness of one of the nurses who allowed me to use a phone from which I called one of our girlfriends. Tamra immediately recognized the gravity of the situation, and came to the hospital and picked me up. She took me to her home where she made me eat while I tried to explain what had happened.

I called Debbie's mother and explained the situation. Virginia sort of understood what I was describing. She had been a nurse her entire working career and in fact still worked as a home care nurse. I explained how the CAT scan showed a tumor and that the neurosurgeon planned to remove it in the morning. She asked, "They aren't planning to do a craniotomy, are they?" When I explained that that was exactly what was planned the seriousness of Debbie's condition finally seeped through her awareness. She wished us luck and asked to be kept informed. I told her I would call throughout the following day as soon as news came available.

It is so good to have friends to rely upon and Tamra helped get me through the longest night of my life. She drove me back to the rental cabin after I had eaten and made the difficult call to Debbie's mother. We retrieved my vehicle and gathered our scattered belongings and unfinished groceries in it. I followed Tamra back to Asheville and somehow managed to drive through the torrent of tears that continued to pour down my face in a flood.

Tamra prepared a bed for me and I lie upon it. There was no sleep for me that night. I tossed and agonized over the shambles my idyllic life had become in a moment's time. Indeed, I have not had a night of peaceful sleep since. Things are good, and then they're not. Two people can be lovingly entwined in peaceful serenity and have that serenity swept away in an instant. Life itself can absent itself in the blink of an eye and no one can do a damn thing about it.

All I knew for sure was that on the morning following our fifth wedding anniversary Debbie woke with the understanding she had been married to me for five full years- and her brain had exploded into shards with that realization.

CHAPTER 10

After my completely sleepless night I was back at the hospital by six in the morning. I went directly to the NICU where Debbie lie sleeping amid the antiseptic smell and constant buzzing and beeping of life monitoring machines. I watched as her heartbeat and respiration caused repeated sine waves to appear on her monitor. The nurse assured me that all was well and that I could waken Debbie, as it was time for her to be prepared for her surgery. Debbie seemed ready for her ordeal. She acknowledged verbally that she knew where she was and why she was there. Of course, Debbie does not remember our meeting the morning of the operation at all.

The nurse informed me that I would now have to leave and continue my vigil in the waiting room. I was told that one of the scrub nurses would come periodically throughout the course of the operation to keep me up to date on the neurosurgeon's progress. I was counseled to expect the operation to last anywhere between six to twelve hours. Debbie was wheeled out to undergo what would be the first of the nearly one hundred Magnetic Resonance Imaging (MRI) scans that she would undergo in the coming years. She would be taken from there directly to the pre-op room where someone shaved her head removing the soft gold hair I adored and whose clean soft aroma had always intoxicated me. The neurosurgeon had examined the MRI and now marked Debbie's bare scalp with the lines he would use to guide him as he opened up her skull and proceeded to expose her brain to the open environment of the operating room atmosphere. The future that Debbie and I had felt was so full of joy just a day and a half before was now hanging on the expertise of a man we had not even met until the previous evening.

Dr. Eric Rhoton is probably a few years younger than both Debbie and I. He is the neurosurgeon who had met our incoming ambulance the night before and it was he who calmly and patiently detailed our options that basically came down to either operating now or operating later. He had a confident demeanor.

You know the phrase, "It's not rocket science and it's not brain surgery." I've used it when attempting a new recipe or when encouraging a student to try something that he believes is too difficult. Well, this was brain surgery and there would not be any room for error. Dr. Rhoton in his calm and professional manner had assured us the night before that the operation was not only necessary but that it would be successful.

He told us that he had done it all before many times and that it is what he does. I was still terrified that morning as the operation began, but I had at the very least placed Debbie in what were the most competent hands available to us.

I retired to the waiting room and waited. The coffee machine received my attention throughout the long day. I could not focus to read any of the magazines that were scattered on the end tables. My head swiveled constantly as I took notice of each and every one of the people who entered and left. My heart jumped every time a doctor or nurse came into the room. Was she the one who would tell me about Debbie? Was everything all right?

By ten that morning, the second of September and the second day of the sixth year of our marriage, several of our friends began to drift in to help me pass the time. Tamra had begun a phone web informing our friends of Debbie's predicament and many of them came by to offer their assistance. I know that I was groggy from lack of sleep and that I was completely and thoroughly emotionally drawn. I'm sure I was less than hospitable yet I could not fail to be impressed with the reaction of our friends who stepped up and offered their love at a time when it was needed most.

Love came in a variety of ways. Hugs, repeated and lingering hugs are the thing I remember most. My coffee cup remained filled throughout the day and I was not the one doing the refilling. Sandwiches, snacks, cookies and candies were being continually thrust at me. One of our friends, who will remain nameless for obvious reasons, took me aside and handed me a packet of hashish. Although I appreciated his sentiment I did not accept it. As has been attributed to Henny Youngman, "What's the most important part of telling a joke? Timing!" It's funny if you say it quickly running all the words together as one. I did appreciate the gift of my friend, but the timing was dead wrong. My head could not consider itself; my thoughts, passions and concerns were focused on the operating room where my wife's head was being dissected.

It wasn't until nearly noon when the scrub nurse first appeared to tell me of the operation's progress. My heart stopped momentarily as she approached. My fear had grown with the passing hours but her first words to me were that everything was proceeding normally. She explained that the craniotomy had begun successfully. A piece of Debbie's skull had been removed safely and that the doctor was beginning the process of removing the tumor and reattaching or resecting the portions of the brain that he would be forced to cut through. The nurse told me she would stop by again when that part of the operation had been completed and that I could expect that to last for several more hours. I thanked her, told her I'd be right there waiting for her next report and turned to our friends who accepted this as the good news that it was. We shared another round of hugs for all as we settled back for the long afternoon.

My memories of that day are vague. I plead the lack of sleep and the pure terror of the situation. I know that friends came and that others appeared as some returned to their own jobs and families as the day progressed. I do remember some time that I spent alone but for most of the day there was someone with me. I will be forever thankful to all those folks who offered their help in time of need. The hours passed. Slowly, but they passed. I still jumped whenever a nurse or doctor entered but I accepted that no news was good news and that as long as I wasn't being told anything bad, then nothing bad was happening.

It was near four in the afternoon when the nurse approached me again. Once again she told me things were routine. The doctor had successfully removed the tumor and was doing the resection of Debbie's brain. How crazy, I thought, that digging in a person's brain and removing deadly tumors can be considered routine but by this time of the day I had already come to my own realization of just what a person must endure. Routine for me right now was summed up in just getting through this day without having to make arrangements for Debbie's funeral.

I settled in for what I hoped would be the quick conclusion of Debbie's operation. I had been aware of some of the other families sitting and waiting while their loved ones underwent some procedure or other. I had commiserated with some, sharing our hard luck stories. We each wished each other the best and offered whatever solace we could. I also noticed that as the day progressed most of these folks had heard good news and had left the waiting room to rejoin their families. Many of them stopped by on their way out of the waiting room to wish me luck and to offer their prayers for Debbie's recovery. This was my first example of the warmth of fellow human beings who find themselves in an overwhelming predicament. As I sit here now and recollect the memories of that nightmarish day I am strengthened by the caring that we offered each other but am saddened that most people do not seem to care about others at all, until they find themselves needing help. The healthy must care for the sick, for indeed sickness will overcome us all.

It was past dinnertime when Dr. Rhoton came to the waiting room. His report was good. Debbie had survived the operation, the tumor was removed from her brain, her skull had been closed up and Debbie was on her way to post-op recovery. I could join Debbie in the post-op room. Dr. Rhoton warned me that Debbie might not be coherent. In fact, he wanted me to engage her in conversation so that I might judge for myself if she was still Debbie or if her trauma had caused irreparable damage. He said that I knew her best and he wanted my opinion.

The doctor had warned me that Debbie might not be fully engaged; he did not warn me about Debbie's appearance. I was shocked.

She looked like the Bride of Frankenstein after a villager's riot. There were eighty-two industrial sized staples running from ear to ear across the top of her skull that had been shaved clean. Lights from the ceiling reflected themselves in the baldness that remained. There were tubes from her nose that were draining blood. There were countless number of leads, wires and connectors linking her to the life support mechanisms that monitored her continuing well being. An oxygen mask was attached to her face and covered her mouth. There were several leads attached to her arm, each one dripping some fluid or other into her body. Other tubes snaked out from beneath her hospital gown and had been inserted in her vagina. I was informed this was a catheter that would drain her urine so that she would not have to rise from the bed in order to pee. She lie on her side in an open in the back hospital gown and most terrifying to me there was a half gallon size plastic bag attached to a plastic tube which was draining blood and pus from within her head and filling like a gory pillow. I went to her and placed my hand around her fingers. They were the only part of Debbie I could reach without disturbing some of the medical equipment. She looked up at me, smiled and she asked me, "Are you all right?"

We spoke a bit. She was in no pain. Mercifully one of the dripping bags contained morphine and it seemed to be working. Debbie appeared to be OK and I expressed that acknowledgement to the doctor who was standing at the head of Debbie's bed. He told me that he would see us in the morning and he left us alone with the nurses who bustled around Debbie while assuring us that all was well.

A nurse brought me a blanket and a pillow and I lie down on the hard floor beside Debbie's bed. I slept beside my wife who had undergone and survived a major brain operation. I was thankful but still apprehensive. My exhaustion overcame me and I slept. I know I was awakened in the night several times by nurses who came to visibly check on Debbie, but I did sleep some. Debbie still has no recollection of this day.

CHAPTER 11

The next three days of Debbie's recovery from surgery went by in a blur. Neither Debbie nor I had spent much time in hospitals before. I hadn't been in one since I broke my wrist when I was sixteen. We had both seen a doctor for routine exams throughout the years but neither of us had ever had an overnight stay before. The hospital is not where I would recommend you spend your next vacation. Granted the patient does receive a very comfortable bed and meals are delivered directly to the bed. Nurses will adjust your angle of incline so that you don't even have to exert yourself in the least to sit up and eat. You are given your own remote control to change the channels on the television at your whim, staff will gently bathe you with sponges dipped in soothing warm water, and you are encouraged to rest. The only problem is that there is no rest in a hospital.

Debbie did sleep for large chunks of her first day recovering from her craniotomy. Her body had endured a major trauma and was exhausted. She would sleep, a half hour would pass, and she would be awakened by a nurse who would ask her how she felt. The inevitable response was tired and the nurse would jot some notes onto the chart at the foot of the bed and Debbie would promptly fall back asleep. The nurses were always kind and gentle but the nature of their job requiring constant monitoring of the recovering post-op patients did cause many visits and interruptions of the rest that Debbie so desperately needed.

As the first day of our new life progressed Debbie slowly became disengaged from some of the cables and wires with which she had become attached. Thankfully for me the bag that had been draining the blood from Debbie's head wound was removed by late afternoon- or about 24 hours after the completion of the surgery. I was so glad to see that go. Its presence crystallized Debbie's vulnerability. The existence of that repository of used up blood reminded me of the fragility of our remaining alive. Its removal was a blessing; a sign that Debbie had mastered her first step toward recovery and that things would and could get better.

During Debbie's cogent moments we were able to talk. I explained to Debbie what had happened. She was still bewildered as to what had occurred. I detailed the time frame since her last memory, her sitting in the rocking chaise on the front porch of the rental cabin. I told her of her surgery and that the doctor had told me we could expect that her recovery time in the hospital could last anywhere between two to six weeks. I primed her for this interlude in our lives.

We visited briefly with some of our friends who came to check on Debbie's prognosis. Mostly, they would peek in, see that Debbie was asleep, and then I would step out and bring them up to date with the latest information I had been given. Everyone who saw Debbie this way, in the first few days following her surgery, remembers the image of a strong, healthy woman laid low. They were all affected and some of them cried. All of them insisted that I could call upon them for anything that we needed. And in the nearly ten years that have followed all of them have kept their word.

I spoke to Debbie of all the phone calls I had made and of all the family and friends who were shaken by her predicament. I had made contact with all of Debbie's family. Her mother had said that she would come to North Carolina to see Debbie just as soon as she could find transportation. Debbie and I agreed that she should wait until a few days more had passed and Debbie would feel a bit stronger.

I can't remember the exact words with which people tried to offer their concern, comfort and love. I'm sorry, we'll pray for you, our thoughts are with you, and so on. There are no proper phrases that will cause healing to a stricken individual. There are no words that can soothe a grieving spouse or place perspective on a sudden trauma. Debbie had been hit by a train. The clichés of kindness that were offered by friends and family were all they had to offer. It was the fact of their words being offered in the grace of kindness and sincerity that made them effective. We were made aware that we were not alone and that people cared. It was enough. Debbie slept, and fell asleep after each and every nurse's interruption of that sleep. I lie beside her on the floor of her hospital room occasionally startling a nurse who entered and was not aware of my presence.

By the second morning following Debbie's surgery it became clear that she would recover from that initial trauma. She became more mobile despite still being tied to various machines. Her arms began waving about slinging wires and tubes in every direction. She began asking questions about the various leads. I turned the monitor that showed the rate of Debbie's respirations and heartbeat so that she could see her own vitality as it presented itself graphically on the screen in continuous patterns of green waves.

Debbie was scratching at her inner thighs. She complained of a rash down there. Her scratching became violent and I became concerned that she could hurt herself or that she might dislodge some of her wiring with her writhing about. I called for a nurse who examined Debbie's legs. There were some scratch marks but no apparent rash had developed. The nurse explained that uncontrollable itching might result from prolonged morphine usage. She said she would inform the doctor of this symptom and that another pain reliever would be substituted in lieu of the morphine that had done its job in keeping Debbie pain free since the surgery. This was accomplished quickly, an exchange of drip bags was completed and Debbie's itching subsided. I was thrilled at the change, as Debbie's attack on herself as caused by the morphine itch had frightened me.

Debbie was served solid food on this day and she completed her hospital provided tray. She asked for and received extra containers of fruit juice that she sipped through a bendable straw. My fear that Debbie's personality had been inalterably changed or lost began to dissipate. She was clearly still my Supergirl. Dr. Rhoton came by twice a day to check on Debbie's condition. He asked Debbie several questions and she answered them with reasonable accuracy. She knew her name. She knew and recognized me. She did not know the exact date but she had the year correct. She was able to lift her limbs upon command, she could wriggle her toes, she could lift her arms and move each individual finger when asked to. She couldn't wriggle her ears when I asked. We weren't upset though as she had never been able to do that before either. She demonstrated her knowledge of current affairs and of her true state of Debbieness when she responded to the query of identifying the President of the United States. Debbie responded, "That bastard!" and I just burst out laughing for the first time in three days. The doctor did require further explanation and Debbie correctly identified President Bush. At that moment everyone present, the doctor, two nurses, Debbie and myself realized that recovery was not far away.

We spent a third day in post-op recovery. The sounds of the hospital had become normal to us. We no longer jumped in fright when a buzzer buzzed or a bell began to ring. We had grown to recognize that these sounds only meant that a nurse would soon appear to change a drip bag or to reset some machine or other. The routine became tiresome to us both. The constant interruption by nurses and doctors who came to monitor and examine Debbie was annoying. We recognized the need for this yet we both longed to be able to sleep for longer than thirty minutes without interruption. Debbie kept trying to get up from the bed. The nurses had asked me to keep Debbie still as she was creating havoc with the leads to her monitors. I explained that I was doing my best. They pleaded with Debbie to remain still and just rest. Debbie would acquiesce, but when the next nurse appeared to visibly check Debbie's vitals Debbie asked her pointedly, "How can I rest when you keep coming here?" The nurse looked at me and I chuckled and said, "See, what I have to live with!"

Sometime in the night of the third day since surgery, and the fourth day since our wedding anniversary, Debbie awoke with a tremendous urge to pee. She began yanking at the cords and wires that attached her to the bed and she actually stood up from the bed. I asked her what she was doing and she told me she had to pee. I endeavored to explain that she was and had been attached to a catheter for the last three days and all she had to do was to lie back down and let it go. She could not comprehend this concept. She insisted she had to pee and she actually squatted down alongside the bed. Her purse had been stashed by her bedside and she was squatting above it and trying to pee in her own purse. Fortunately, the buzzing caused by her ripping out some of her leads brought a nurse to the room. Upon seeing Debbie out of the bed and ridiculously trying to urinate into her own purse the nurse seized Debbie and set her back upon the bed. The nurse patiently explained the presence and purpose of the catheter tubing and Debbie returned to sleep. The nurse wrote several things on the chart and left us to our slumber.

The next morning Dr. Rhoton came by once more. He questioned Debbie and once again ran through the series of commands to move various parts of her body. Debbie obviously passed all these neurological exams and the doctor then surprised us by telling us that we would be released to go home that afternoon. I was flabbergasted. Just a few days earlier he had told me to expect a hospital stay that could easily last a month and here we were being discharged after just three days of post-op recovery. The doctor insisted that we could be discharged safely and he set up an appointment to see him in his Asheville office on September 10th at which time we would discover the results of the pathology exams that had been performed on the excised tumor. Until then, we were encouraged to allow Debbie as much rest and comfort as she could handle. The doctor explained that the tumor might be either malignant or benign. Should it be benign, Debbie's full recovery would be pretty much assured. Should it be malignant then we would discuss treatment options at our visit.

I called our respective mothers and asked them to pass on the good news that we were going home. Debbie's mom said she would join us in a day and urged us to be careful and to take care. I wished her a safe journey and that I appreciated her upcoming assistance.

And that was that. The nightmare of Debbie's seizure, subsequent ambulance rides, her emergency surgery and removal of a potentially fatal brain tumor had been completed. We were going home, to our own bed, to our pets D.D. the Dog and C.C. the Cat, to our partially completed home extension, and to a new life that we didn't quite yet fully understand.

I wondered then, as I still wonder now, as to why Debbie had been released from the hospital so soon. I was glad as we were much more comfortable without the bustle of the hospital all about us, but still, why had Debbie been released so soon? I have come to believe that it is partially because Debbie proved herself to be a troublesome patient once she awakened from the drugs that had kept her sedated through the pain and trauma of surgery. Her tossing and turning and her constant desire to rise from the bed did make the lives of her nurses troublesome. I'm sure that the scene of her trying to pee in her purse had impressed the nursing staff with Debbie's intolerance of further bed restrictions. But mostly, the reason I have come to believe that Debbie was released so quickly was that the hospital still had no proof of Debbie's insurance coverage. You will recall that I had not had time to gather my belongings or wallet when the ambulance took us to the hospital. I believe that the doctor was pressured to release Debbie in order to make room for an incoming patient that the hospital knew had coverage and would therefore be more lucrative. Maybe I'm right, maybe I'm wrong. I'll never know for sure, but at the time I was just thrilled to get Debbie out of the hospital and back home.

Our drive back up the mountain was uneventful. We arrived home and Debbie was comfortably set up in bed with no wires or cables to hinder her movements. She was able to get up, stand, walk about and use the toilet without assistance. We spent a good portion of the evening answering phone calls from friends who had come by to see us in the hospital and had been told we were discharged. Everyone was thrilled and surprised, none more than me.

To this day, Debbie still has no recollection of these events.

CHAPTER 12

We returned home to a house in disarray. Debbie and I had finally scraped together enough cash to hire a contractor to build an extension onto our home. We had designed a living room that would extend from what would become the former entrance to the home. The room would have large windows on three sides that would allow us to enjoy the view of the Dutch Creek valley. At the time of Debbie's seizure the new room had been closed in from the elements but had not yet been dry walled. Tools and loose nails were strewn all about haphazardly and it was an obstacle course to get from our new front entrance back to the older portion of the house where our bedroom is.

The contractor met us as we drove up our drive. He had graciously agreed to feed our dog and cat during our weekend anniversary getaway. I had arranged with him beforehand and he had maintained the secret of our anniversary trip from Debbie. When the drastic and unexpected events of the weekend transpired I had called him to ask if he could continue to watch D.D. and C.C. during what was bound to become a prolonged absence. He did not believe me when I told him of Debbie's seizure and her upcoming operation.

We had worked closely with the contractor once we had agreed to have him do the work for us. It was as if we had a daily houseguest. We made a great effort to ensure that he was happy in his work place. We played the music he liked to hear and made sure he realized that he could work at a comfortable pace, raid our refrigerator at will or bring his son to work with him if he needed to help his wife with child care chores. He was convinced that we had just chosen to remain on vacation an extra week or so and although he was willing to accept responsibility for our animals he just would not accept that Debbie had been stricken. The poor fellow turned white as a sheet when I helped Debbie step out of our car. Debbie still had the staples aligned across her bald scalp and there was no longer any talk of a phantom excuse to extend our vacation. For the next several months until the completion of the construction project our house was filled daily with the sounds of hammers and power saws. It may not have been the ideal location for a recovering patient, but it was ours and we were glad to be there and to begin enjoying the extended views from our semi-completed new living room.

Our animals were delighted to see us. D.D. the Dog jumped about in a tizzy but did seem a bit confused by Debbie's apparent weakness and change in temperament. Debbie did not take the dog in her lap as she had used to. D.D. still remained loyal and in fact took it upon herself to become overly protective of Debbie during this time. The dog stayed at Debbie's feet and followed her as she maneuvered her way from room to room. It was as if D.D. could sense that Debbie needed a little extra love and care at this time.

We had gotten D.D. about a year and a half before. She had been the runt of a litter of nine dogs that had been whelped by a mutt that belonged to a friend of ours. The mother was a wiry, black hound of sorts; the father was unknown. We went to see the puppies when they were just a few weeks old and had not yet been weaned. The puppies were mixed in color. Three were all black, three were all white and a couple were both black and white at the same time. These eight puppies all jumped up and stormed the fence of their enclosure when we approached. One smaller puppy, all red, just stood back from the others, sat and looked peacefully at us as we opened the fence and entered the cage. Debbie had insisted that we finally replace the dogs of our beloved memory that had passed and although I was not sure I wanted to, I agreed that we would accept one of the puppies from this litter. I chose the quiet little red one. Neither Debbie nor I ever regretted that choice as that quiet little runt grew to be the most loyal and protective dog that either of had ever had. We drove home that day with the puppy on my lap. The dog had never been in a car before and the curving mountain roads did not yet agree with her. She puked in my lap and our bonding was complete.

We already had C.C. She was already eleven years old, had been named by Debbie as a tribute to the song C.C. Rider, and one of the reasons we had hesitated obtaining a new dog was that we were unsure of how that new dog would relate to our already elderly cat. The two met, the dog cautiously approached the cat and tried to lick her. The cat gently swiped the dog's nose and they were friends forever. Our worries were needless. All we needed to do now was to name our new dog. We spent an hour or two trying out different and highly forgettable names. I can't remember a single one. Then it came to me. I hadn't wanted a dog in the first place. This puppy was to be Debbie's dog. D.D.! Debbie's Dog! Our family was complete what with C.C. who now became known as C.C. the Cat and our new puppy, D.D. who instantly became D.D. the Dog. Debbie's Dog the Dog! We knew it was redundant but within seconds of her christening both Debbie and I were already singing out the name D.D. the Dog to the melody of Beethoven's fifth symphony. D. D. the Dog, it sounded so good, and it just seemed to fit.

C.C. was never so demonstrative as the dog but also somehow recognized some sort of change in Debbie. The cat would sleep with Debbie in the bed and would consistently fall off to sleep in Debbie's lap. Both the animals seemed to respond to Debbie's new instability with a bit of extra gentleness.

Debbie's brother Brad arrived the day after we had returned home with Debbie's mom. Virginia immediately went into her home nursing mode. She examined Debbie thoroughly taking close looks at the incisions that had been made in her skull. Virginia seemed to think everything had gone all right and she then proceeded to take over the kitchen and began preparing sandwiches for everyone. We were glad to have her there, as I know she was glad to see Debbie and to see for herself that she had survived. I didn't mind the company but I insisted that she allow us to treat her as a guest in our home and not as a nurse or maid. Virginia is and has always been a competent and an in charge person. Debbie's streak of stubbornness and her desire to do things her own way certainly was inherited from her mom.

We passed the next few days quietly. Debbie was mostly resting, but also spending much of the day with her mom and brother and catching up on family news. There was quite a bit of television watching going on while I took care of the logistics of shopping, cleaning, cooking and rearranging my work schedule and informing my landscape clients of our emergency. Most were quite understanding and rescheduled my missed appointments.

One lady, however, was completely bent out of shape that I had not been available to mow her lawn the previous morning. I apologized and tried to explain that my wife had suffered a brain tumor and undergone emergency surgery. All she cared about was her damn lawn. I explained that I could be by the very next morning but she was insistent that I compensate her for the unmowed lawn. She wanted me to come by and not charge her for my time. I told her she could go "F" herself. I did not then, nor do I now, regret having lost that client. She became the first I have seen of the many cold-hearted individuals who were so hung up in the minutiae of their own lives that they could not see the needs and problems of their fellow humans. I have been stunned over the last ten years by our country's shift from caring about our neighbors to the heartlessness and greed that now seems to permeate to the core of our political values.

Debbie and I, of course, did have some other fish to fry. We knew that Debbie would be unable to return to her position as the horticulturalist and manager of the hundreds of flowerbeds at the local golf and country club where she worked. We arranged for Debbie to be placed on a leave of absence. We assured her employers that we would keep them up to date on Debbie's recovery and that it was Debbie's intent to return to work in the spring as soon as the doctors cleared her for work. Debbie's employers did respond magnificently. They arranged for the hat to be passed and we were presented with a cash bonus to help tide us over through the oncoming winter.

I returned to work myself knowing that Debbie's mom and brother were present to care for Debbie should she need any assistance. I mowed lawns, deadheaded flowers, cleared weeds and deadfalls, blew leaves off driveways and continued the maintenance of the yards that people had entrusted to my care. My mind was elsewhere though. I could not stop wondering about what would be the word concerning the pathology on Debbie's tumor. She seemed fine; her recovery from the surgery was swift and relatively pain free and uneventful. Did that mean the tumor was benign? God knows I certainly hoped so.

Debbie and I did not discuss the upcoming appointment. We never spoke about our desire that the tumor be judged benign. That was understood and we went through these days of recovery and waiting with the expectation that we would be fine and that we would continue to live life as we had. We maintained the illusion that all was well. We told folks of the upcoming appointment to be held on the 10th of the month at which time we would be told Debbie's diagnosis. I expected that the report would be favorable and just never really considered the alternative.

Virginia accompanied us on our visit to the neurosurgeon's offices in Asheville. We did what I have come to recognize as the doctor's office waltz. We waited with others in a reception area and were then after a while called up front where we were directed to a small examination room at which time we began to wait anew. We examined the diplomas and certificates that were displayed on the wall. Dr. Rhoton did have a medical degree and seemed to be highly recognized by his peers among neurosurgeons. Finally, the doctor joined us.

Debbie was fully examined. The doctor carefully checked the staples that were still binding Debbie's head together and told us everything looked fine and that the staples would be able to be removed by the end of the month.

He then told us the results of the pathology report. The doctor told us that the tumor was a malignancy. It was a form of brain cancer called an anaplastic astrocytoma. The doctor described the shape of the cancerous cells as star shaped, hence the name astrocytoma. He said that this was a Level or Grade III tumor and could be expected to reappear if it was not treated. He explained that although he had removed the majority of the tumorous material that it was impossible to remove all the microscopic bits of tumor that had embedded themselves in Debbie's brain. The doctor explained that in his opinion the best course of further treatment would be to have Debbie begin an extreme regimen of both chemotherapy and radiation treatments to kill and destroy the remaining tumor fragments. The doctor further explained that in some ways this was a fortunate tumor as it would not metastasize or move about the body. It was malignant and it would continue to grow and cause life threatening issues if not treated, but that it would remain located in the same spot and should therefore be a bit easier to treat and to monitor. He suggested we involve our local hospital in these procedures so that we would not have to travel as much to begin and maintain treatment. I remember that he asked if we had any questions. I don't remember that we did other than to arrange the logistics of setting up appointments with our local oncologists.

We never did ask, nor did the doctor offer any information about potential life expectancies. We understood that we would follow through on whatever treatments were recommended to us and that our life would continue. We would continue. Debbie and I were in love and I would not leave her side.

September 1st, and Debbie's seizure had led through an emergency craniotomy on the 2nd, recovery in the hospital until the 5th, a few days more of home rest and recovery, and a malignant pathology report on the 10th. These were the ten days that shook our world. The rest of the world caught up with us the following morning.

CHAPTER 13

Some times I just want to beat somebody with a stick. I want to shake them and force some compassion into their bodies. I want to move them from their self-centered universe and bring them forth forcefully to witness the suffering of the rest of the world. I know that feeling this way is counter productive to my own well being but I cannot deny the anger that controls me when I am faced with inane and insipid bureaucratic rules.

Here is my current case in point. For nearly ten years now Debbie has been forced to undergo MRI scans. Depending on the varying nature of the activity inside her brain the MRI's have sometimes been scheduled as frequently as once a month. In the last year, however, Debbie has not faced any extraordinary crisis points and the schedule of her MRI's has been set at just two scans a year. This is a wonderful thing and shows that Debbie's condition has finally stabilized after all these years. In the meantime, however, Debbie has undergone close to a hundred different MRI scans. Almost all of these scans have been administered by our local hospital system. We are there so often that the MRI technicians have become our friends and they share photos of their growing families with us. One technician, in fact, was so distraught she was transferring to another job with a local orthopedist that she called us at home one afternoon to let us know personally of her job transfer. She did not want us to wonder where she had gone and took the added step of calling. She is an angel and we will never forget her kindness and warmth.

Anyway, for nearly ten years now I have been able to receive the MRI order from Debbie's doctor and then using that order have been able to call the MRI scheduling department and place Debbie's name upon the schedule. Today, I called the scheduling office and was told that I must appear in person with the doctor's order before they could place Debbie on the schedule. I have never had to do that before. I would order the MRI, we would appear on time, and I would give the order to the technicians when we arrived. I explained to the woman on the other end of my phone that Debbie had been following the same procedure for nearly ten years now and I wished to know why the procedure needed to be changed. Must I leave Debbie while I made a separate and unnecessary trip to town?

It was acknowledged that Debbie's record of her numerous previous MRI's was current and that the office had the contact information for Debbie's doctors. Still, there was an adamant refusal to schedule Debbie until they had the order form in their own greedy, grubby hands. No real reason was given me for the change in scheduling policy. All I was given was a repeated refusal to continue scheduling over the phone and the bottom line is that I was unable to schedule Debbie's next MRI. Now I will have to make a separate trip to the hospital and schedule in person.

Now this, quite honestly, just ticks me off. The hospital is a service provider. The hospital provides service for those who are sick or otherwise in need of medical care. Debbie, being a brain cancer patient, is sick and in need of the hospital's services. Furthermore, the nature of Debbie's illness prevents her from competently handling her own scheduling and I as her husband and legally assigned agent must take care of these chores for her. I guarantee that there is nobody in the world who would choose to have brain cancer and be forced to endure the indignities that the cancer has caused. In other words, sick people are just that; they are people who are sick and in need of assistance. Is it too much to ask that the hospital provide a small courtesy to its patients by allowing them to continue what has worked for ten years or must the patients accommodate a procedure that has no reason for its existence? Basically, it boils down to this- a phone call was all I ever needed to make so why must I now appear in person?

It's a matter of dignity. Every time the hospital creates a situation in which the patient or caregiver is placed in the role of supplicant for services then a small bit of our dignity as a human being is diminished. Sick people should never be placed in the role of pleading for a treatment or a service that their doctor has prescribed. Doctors should be ruling the health care system but they do not. Increasingly we have come to rely upon bureaucrats and insurance salesmen to determine what are and aren't acceptable policies and treatments. This is shameful because of the way it encourages us to demean the experiences and needs of those who have become ill.

I believe that the policies of our health care systems must serve this population of sick people. Their employees, their office procedures, their billing and financial offices must cater to the special needs of this population. Sick people, or the families of those sick, should not have to be caused any unnecessary discomfort. The sick and their families are already overburdened with the trials of caring for their loved one. The needs of a bureaucrat are low on our priority lists and that is the way it should be. The compassion for our fellow humans demands this. Sadly, I have come to discover, in some instances the bureaucrats rule. So, thank you, beautiful lady who I just got off the phone with! You have created and followed an unnecessary rule and you have made my life just a wee tinge more difficult. As if!

Yes, there are times I just wish I could beat somebody with a stick!

CHAPTER 14

Some days because of their incredible shock value of events become completely memorable to all who have lived to see them. The ten days of September 1st through September 10th, 2001 are memorable to Debbie and I because of the devastating attack on Debbie's brain caused by a cancerous tumor. The morning of September 11th is remembered because of a stunning, shocking and devastating attack upon our country. I would wager that if you were at least five years old on that morning you remember where you were when you either saw or heard about the planes that flew directly into the twin towers of the World Trade Center in New York City causing them to collapse in a fiery inferno.

Debbie and I had returned home from our meeting with the neurosurgeon the previous afternoon. Debbie's mom, Virginia, was with us. We had spent the evening discussing and preparing for the long struggle we were about to face. Debbie's tumor was not benign. It was malignant. It was cancer.

Debbie accepted this fate with her customary peaceful calm. She did not shed a tear. I cried enough for us both. Debbie's concerns were centered more upon the time and travel requirements of her upcoming treatments. Dr. Rhoton had recommended both chemotherapy and radiation treatments in his plan to fight off Debbie's cancer. Debbie without hesitation had agreed to undergo any potential treatments that would save her life. She understood that the treatments should begin as soon as we could arrange them and that the side effects of the treatments would be debilitating and that she would require special help from me as they progressed. We both accepted our fate. Debbie would undergo the medical procedures with calm and courage and I would provide whatever logistical assistance was necessary. I would become cook, chauffeur, laundress, maid and be unwavering in my support of my wife. I joked that when these months of therapies were complete that I would have developed the skills necessary to make someone a good wife. By the way, I believe I have.

I had arranged several work related appointments the morning of the 11th. I had risen early and prepared breakfast for Debbie, Virginia and myself. My first meeting with a client was set for quarter to ten and I had gathered all my necessary tools into the back of our pickup and was preparing to leave the house. Virginia had assured me that Debbie would be well cared for and that I need not worry even though I wouldn't expect to be home until dark. I was literally walking out the door when the phone rang.

Our friend Mike was calling from Colorado. Mike had been the fellow who introduced Debbie and I years ago and although he and his girlfriend, also named Debbie, had moved away to be closer to Debbie's sister we still remained in close contact. Mike had been informed of Debbie's seizure and subsequent surgery and had been aware of our visit to the neurosurgeon the day before. I just assumed that Mike wanted to know the result of that visit and I began to tell him about the cancerous diagnosis we had been given.

"Turn on your TV", Mike screamed across the phone lines.

"Don't you want to know about Debbie?"

"Yes, but TURN ON YOUR TV!"

I flipped on the television and was greeted with a view of the World Trade Center. This was a building I had no problem recognizing on sight. I had grown up in Brooklyn and had seen the construction of the towers from their beginnings. Along with millions of other New Yorkers I marveled as the construction grew larger and higher with the passing weeks. At least several times a week I entered Manhattan driving along the Brooklyn-Queens Expressway (BQE) and crossing over the Brooklyn Bridge. The new towers dominated the view of New York harbor and their appearance changed the cityscape drastically.

It took a few seconds for me to realize that one of the towers was ablaze. The commentator had mentioned something about an attack. I called to Debbie and to Virginia to join me and see what was going on. They had barely made it in front of the screen when we watched horrorifically as a plane seemed to arrive from nowhere and sped directly into the second tower exploding in a puffball of flame. What the hell was that?

In the next few moments we saw the replay of that moment shown over and over again. Immediately my thoughts went in the direction of my hometown. God forbid that any of my sisters or their kids were in the area that morning. My sister Audrey did work in the city occasionally when her work as an audio technician for NBC demanded it. Roberta, Audrey's twin, usually stayed in Brooklyn, but what of the kids? I had Mike on the phone still and told him of Debbie's diagnosis. He expressed his best wishes and concern but understood when I told him I had to try to call my family in the city.

I couldn't get through to Roberta. I did reach Audrey in her home in New Jersey. She was fine and she told me that she would continue trying Roberta and we then spoke about Debbie's diagnosis. How strange it seemed to me that the discussion of my wife's newly discovered cancer should be relegated to such a secondary role in our conversation.

There was nothing more I could do. I placed an American flag on the table near our front door and I went on to work. I spent the day on my hands and knees weeding out flowerbeds. I worked in a complete daze, my hands and fingers continued to operate efficiently as I worked my way from one bed to another, but my mind was scattered and worried. My wife had brain cancer and my hometown had been attacked and people were dead. It was too much for me to get my head around and many a flower that day received extra watering from my tears.

My family was safe. Everyone was accounted for, if not necessarily present. My nephew, Eric, had been attending at Stuyvesant High School. His school was only a few blocks from what the commentators were very quickly calling ground zero. The students had been dismissed almost immediately and became eyewitnesses to the burning and subsequent collapse of the two towers. Eric was unable to find transportation back into Brooklyn as subway service had been halted. He stayed the night with a classmate who lived in Manhattan and they walked together to that friend's home. A few days later Eric related to me that he had seen people jumping to their deaths from the higher levels of the towers. There was nothing I could say.

I grieved for the loss of life along with my countrymen. I displayed the flag proudly and with recognition of the fact that on this day our country had united in a way not seen in my lifetime. I had not been asked to wave my flag. I just did. It seemed the right thing to do.

The week following 9/11 was a busy time for Debbie and I. It was clear that Debbie was recovering quickly from her traumatic surgery. We became able to go out for short walks when I returned from work each day. I had called the oncology center at our local hospital and appointments had been made for Debbie to meet with both a medical and a radiation oncologist. We learned that the medical oncologist would prescribe and administer the chemotherapy program and that the radiation oncologist would set the parameters for and administer the radiation treatments.

We met with a social worker who arranged to have Debbie create a living will and to have me assigned as her legal agent. We met in a room that was being used to administer chemotherapy treatments to a number of patients. They were reclining as drip bags attached to their arms slowly dosed out the poison that was hoped to combat their cancers. One couple, a few years older than we, needed witnesses to a will they were creating. Debbie and I added our names to their document and swore that we had seen them sign it themselves. The four of us spoke a few moments. They told us that the illness had brought them closer together as a couple and that they were not afraid. We took great comfort in meeting them. These two exuded a courage in the face of adversity that I could use. Debbie, of course, had been nothing but the personification of strength and will from the beginning.

It was determined that we would fight Debbie's tumor with all the means that were available to us. Debbie would begin a chemotherapy regimen. She was fortunate, that is, if a recently diagnosed cancer patient can be deemed to be fortunate. Her chemotherapy would not have to be administered through a drip bag. She would be able to take her chemotherapy in an oral form; a series of pills she could take orally. Debbie would not have to lie for hours while the bags dripped slowly into her veins. It was agreed that the type of medication would change each month, thereby doubling the chances that one of the medications would be effective. Research had shown that drip type chemotherapy was ineffective in crossing the blood-brain barrier. The pills, it was hoped, would effectively travel to the brain where they would hopefully begin to specifically attack the tumorous cells that remained following surgery.

The doctor wrote a prescription for the pills and I went across the street to the pharmacy to obtain them. The script had been written for a month and the pharmacist returned with two pills and presented me with a bill for four thousand dollars. I choked. We did not have four thousand dollars and two pills was just the dosage required for the first day. I was told that Debbie's insurance would not cover the cost of the prescribed chemotherapy. This became the first of several instances where insurance refused to honor the specifics of our doctor's instructions. It was the opinion of the insurance company that a cheaper method of chemotherapy should be employed. I would not argue that cheaper methods of curing might not be warranted, but, the doctors had just explained to us that because of the nature of the blood-brain barrier, the prescribed method of treatment was the only one felt to have a real chance of destroying Debbie's tumor and allowing her to go on with her life. The insurance company would have gladly paid for a cheaper and less efficacious manner of treatment and the result would have been Debbie's death. How is that compassionate or cost effective?

I returned to the hospital and waited while the doctor made several phone calls. The insurance people acquiesced and finally agreed that they were obligated to pay for whatever the doctor felt most assured Debbie's continued survival. Of course, had I not been appalled by their refusal to pay and had the doctor not insisted upon the course of treatment he had prescribed, Debbie would have died as a result of insurance negligence.

My vibrant and beautiful wife had been stricken with brain cancer. The twin towers had been attacked by suicide terrorists and the towers weakened and demolished, fell. Debbie had been laid low, quivering like a bowl of jelly in spastic seizures. A program of destroying Debbie's tumor was underway. Chemotherapy and radiation would be applied directly against the tumor and it would hopefully be sufficient in saving her life. Would that our country had instituted a direct attack upon those who had attacked us. The attack on the World Trade Center was a criminal case of mass murder. We ignored the culprits and instead we began a campaign against the country of Iraq. The Iraqis had no terrorists on board the doomed planes and no evidence existed that Iraq had planned or cooperated in the planning and implementation of the 9/11 attacks. Debbie was at war with the brain tumor that had attacked her and having gathered the best possible advice proceeded with a plan to fight her tumor. Our country responded quickly, but not against those who had actually attacked us. We began a war but chose the wrong enemy. It was comparable to Debbie appearing at the hospital having seizures, discovering the cause of the seizures was a tumor, and then proceeding to treat her for a broken leg.

By the end of September I had removed the American flag from the threshold of our home. My love for my fellow Americans has never weakened but I could not support the policy of declaring war on those who were innocent.

CHAPTER 15

Debbie and I began to settle into our new reality and that included the fact that Debbie was now a walking time bomb and that things inside her head could choose to explode and take her consciousness and her life at any moment. Of course, this is potentially true for any and all of us, and it is true for us all at any time whatsoever. Fortunately, most of us do not dwell on the fact of our impending demise. We just go about our daily routines. Debbie and I proceeded to go about our daily routines, but I admit that from day one of this journey, I always wondered about what was going on inside my wife's head. I'm not sure that makes me much different from the other billions of husbands in the world but I do know I was focused.

Debbie's job in the fall of 2001 was to regain her strength and to endure the trials of undergoing her chemotherapy and radiation regimens. It was understood she would be unable to work for at least six months. The doctor had explained that Debbie's driving privileges were automatically suspended because of her presentation with a seizure. It would be quite a disaster were someone suspect to seizures be behind the wheel of a vehicle and we were quite willing to allow the required time to pass and to give a chance for the anti-seizure medications Debbie had been placed on to become effective. To this day, Debbie has not had a second seizure. Obviously one was enough.

Debbie has held only two jobs since her early twenties. Both were in the field of landscaping and horticulture maintenance. The first was with a landscaping firm in Raleigh. Debbie worked for those folks for nineteen years and would easily have continued with them for an additional nineteen years had she not chosen (finally!) to fall in love with and subsequently move up the mountain to live with me. The second job was with a local country club and golf course just a twenty minute ride from our home. In both locations Debbie had began as a crew worker and in each position she worked her way up the ladder and became a crew leader and manager. Debbie's work ethic was impeccable. She was always on time, her flowerbeds were immaculately kept, her crews were kept busy throughout the seasons and her designs were acknowledged by one and all to be fabulous.

The nature of Debbie's work required her to be healthy, strong and able to drive motor vehicles. She spent hours daily in the dirt first teaching and then working alongside the crews of Mexican migrants assigned to her. Her career had been shortstopped by the tumor. We hoped she would be able to return in the upcoming spring but we had no assurances that would or could occur. The administrators of the country club placed Debbie on the rolls of those who are temporarily unemployed. They agreed that Debbie could return to work as soon as the doctor's cleared her to do so. She was presented with a cash bonus that helped us through that first fall.

At the time of Debbie's tumor I was also working as a landscaper. I had not put in the twenty five years plus that Debbie had, but I did have the advantage of Debbie managing my work and making sure I was trained correctly in the things that I did. With Debbie's help I had accumulated a client list of nearly twenty families and I worked hard to maintain their yards and their trust. There were times when I found the peaceful serendipity that can be afforded to those who work outdoors, but mostly I found the work to be difficult and dirty. I came home a muddy mess and began to cherish the time I could spend in the shower at the end of a workday allowing the hot water to soothe the muscles in my aging back and washing the dirt and sweat off my body.

Most of my previous working career had been spent indoors. Disregarding the many years I spent working with my father at the gas station in Brooklyn, and the summers I spent as a teen as a camp counselor, every other job I had ever held was performed mostly indoors. I had owned and managed my own business for nearly a decade, I had been a children's librarian for several years and I had been a retail salesman and store manager for a nationally known chain store.

In the late eighties I became burned out running my business. I had successfully operated a balloon delivery service. I would dress up in any costume the customer desired and I would make an appearance at birthday parties singing songs, telling stories and playing my kazoo. I hired students from our local college to join me as many folks were interested in presenting their friends a balloon bouquet delivered by a young lady in a sexy outfit and as cute as I am, I just did not fit the bill. I appreciated the independence working for myself afforded and I certainly relished the opportunity to take a month off at a time whenever I wished. All it required was the hiring and training of a trustworthy helper. I had no problems hiring folks. Many of my friends volunteered their time just to have the opportunity to say had been a belly-dancing gorilla at a sorority party. It was fun. After doing it for ten years though, the novelty of the whole thing wore off for me and I came to realize that the part of the job I liked the best were the times I performed at children's parties and was able to entertain them with my storytelling. This feeling meshed with the satisfaction I had enjoyed as a camp counselor and I realized my future should allow me the opportunity to work with young children.

I began attending classes at Appalachian State University with the intention of earning my college degree and a state license to teach. I maintained the balloon shop and used the money I earned from it to pay my tuition. Upon graduation I obtained employment in rural Georgia where I served as a grade school teacher for three years. They were interesting years in that I was the only white male in the school in which I taught. It astonished me that after just a few hours that first morning how comfortable I felt. Kids are just kids; I accepted them and they accepted me.

I left Georgia because although I had successfully led my students through the learning of their three "R's" the administrators considered me a troublemaker. They may have been right.

At one point in my third year one of my students had asked me why it was that he and many of his classmates were forced to ride the school bus to our rural school when they lived in town where another school was located. I did not know and told the student I would attempt to find out. I found out all right. The district in which I worked was arbitrarily bussing black children so that the school in town would remain mostly white. This to me was unconscionable. The entire purpose of bussing was to create long term racial harmony by forcing the disparate members of our society to interact with one another. My own childhood had been spent in multi-racial neighborhoods and schools and this background allowed me the ability to deal fairly and effectively with anyone. These children, my students, were being forced to ride an extra forty-five minutes on the bus twice a day to help perpetuate what is an antiquated system of enforced separation of people.

Well, I found these things out and I was shocked I had been blind to the situation for the three years I had worked there. I just assumed the students being delivered to my classroom were the ones who lived in the outlying farmlands surrounding our school building. The crap hit the fan when I informed my students of my discovery and they in turn told their respective mothers. It wasn't long after that I was called in to see my principal who told me my contract would not be renewed and I would have to find another place to teach the coming semester. The principal told me I was a good teacher, my students had and were doing well on their standardized exams but that the members of the community (the whites, I assume) could not figure me out. He told me, "Mr. Block, you're not one of us and you're not one of them either!" I have come to cherish the truth in that statement and have always continued to try to see the larger picture whenever any issue presents itself.

I found myself returning to the mountains of the Blue Ridge and obtained employment first as a teaching assistant at a local high school and then as a social worker working with children who had been adjudicated as violent and were in desperate need of mentoring and a positive male role model. I enjoyed this work and it was this job I was engaged in when Debbie and I married in 1996.

By the end of the millennium the bureaucracy of social work grew tired of me. The kids loved me as I would always advocate in their favor and they could count on my word. My administrators, once again, found me suspect because I would fight tooth and nail for every benefit the law afforded the children entrusted to my care. I was released just prior to my becoming vested in the pension system to which I had been contributing a portion of my salary. As it turns out, my bosses had erred in their arithmetic. I had accumulated enough time on the job, and after a labor hearing I did receive a lump sum payout upon my dismissal. I used some of this money to purchase equipment and began to work the landscaping business I was engaged in when Debbie's tumor struck.

I have bothered you, dear reader, with a synopsis of our work history to illuminate the fact that both Debbie and I were and are working people. We paid our taxes; we contributed to the Social Security system and never had gotten into trouble with the law. We had health insurance that we had obtained through Debbie's employer. We are not beggars; we are just a married couple who fate has chosen to test by having Debbie be the victim of a brain tumor. What has happened to us can and does happen to good people every day. We are you and you are we.

CHAPTER 16

Ladies and gentlemen, have you ever just wished that you could lose some of that unwanted weight? Have you ever imagined that the pounds would just melt away? Could you ever have conceived that you could become skinny without having to torment yourself to hours of sweaty exercise and workouts? Can you believe that all this can be done without ever even having to leave the comfort of your own easy chair? You, yes, even you, can lose that unwanted poundage by taking just two pills a day. Your weight loss is guaranteed! This program is 100% effective- you will lose weight! And not just a measly pound or two, you will be amazed as the flesh seemingly melts off you body as snow melts in the sunshine. Do you want to be 10, 20, 30, 40; even 50 pounds lighter than you are now? Not satisfied yet? Would you care to discard one quarter to one third of your current body weight while you continue to eat everything that is placed before you? That's right- no diet or exercise required! Sit on your ass, watch television, eat chocolates and ice cream sundaes all day long, and still lose those pounds! Skeptical, you say? Oh, ye of such little faith in the wonders of chemistry! Do you really, really want to lose those pounds? Then stop hesitating, run to your nearest oncologist and beg to be placed on the miraculous (cue the trumpet blasts) Chemotherapy Diet!

Debbie always looked good to me and may have never looked so good as she did to me the long celebratory night of our fifth anniversary. Some may have considered her to be a tinge overweight, but I always felt she was perfect. Debbie weighed 160 pounds at the time of her surgery. She actually had gained a few pounds in the month of her recovery. Not working and being fed constantly to renew her strength had her at 165 when she began the chemotherapy regimen. In the next six months Debbie began shedding weight like it had gone out of style. She dipped below 150 within a month of having begun the pills and continued to lose weight continuously for the next six months. I admit, that for the two to three weeks that Debbie weighed between 115 and 125 I thought I was married to a fashion model. Albeit, one of those strange looking models seen in teen fashion magazines. Her baldness while disconcerting at first was not necessarily without its components of sexiness.

A quick word about Debbie's baldness. It was my intention to allow Debbie anything that would help her feel more comfortable with the changes in her appearance. The first thing almost everyone asked us, was about the regrowth of Debbie's hair. It did grow back eventually except for the front, right quadrant of her scalp where radiation treatments made collateral damage of Debbie's roots on their way to destroying the tumorous remains in her head. Debbie's mother and I agreed that Debbie should have the opportunity to purchase a wig or two and Debbie's mom insisted that this be her gift to us. We went wig shopping and Debbie did choose a couple. In the nearly ten years since her surgery she has not worn the wigs at all. Debbie does wear a baseball cap constantly when she goes outdoors and most people are completely unaware that a full quarter of Debbie's scalp is completely bald and shiny.

Funny thing about the chemotherapy diet, you lose weight, but you will continue to lose weight long after you have reached that ideal weight you had dreamed about. Your spouse and friends will admire your "new you" initially but will watch in horror as weight continues to drop off and ribs begin to stick out. No amount of eating will stop this weight loss as long as you remain on the chemotherapy. Debbie's weight bottomed out at below one hundred pounds, a loss of nearly seventy pounds, or more than one third of her body weight. This, it should be obvious, is not healthy.

Chemotherapy works on the theory that the way to destroy the cancer cells is to poison them. Chemotherapy is poison; doled out in small enough doses that will kill cancer cells but that will not kill the patient. It is a thin line and oncologists will monitor and tweak dosages as necessary but the bottom line is a chemotherapy patient is ingesting poison into their system. The problem is that no chemotherapy exists that will attack only cancer cells and leave the rest of the patient alone. So, poison it is.

There are, of course, other side effects that are caused by the ingestion of poison into one's body. Nausea and vomiting can be so frequent that additional medicines are required to help control the digestive system and even with that additional assistance you can expect that a chemotherapy patient will have fits of uncontrollable vomiting. Debbie's first episode occurred the very first evening within an hour of her taking the pill. By the end of the first week we had stopped counting the number of times Debbie had to run to the nearest sink or commode to allow herself to purge.

One night I had prepared Debbie a special dinner. I had splurged at the grocery and had purchased an expensive cut of steak. I prepared a salad, baked a potato and grilled the steak to medium rare perfection. I was proud of myself as I placed this feast before Debbie. She did not even have a chance to lift her fork when she promptly began to hurl all over the plate. These actions were completely uncontrollable. Dinner was ruined and I was disappointed that Debbie had been unable to eat.

Another time I treated Debbie by taking her out for breakfast. We were sharing a pot of coffee and all was good. Then the waitress slid a fresh omelet in front of Debbie. Debbie, almost casually, leaned over her plate and proceeded to douse her omelet with a vomitous sauce. I hurriedly threw some cash on the table, grabbed some napkins, and got Debbie out of there before the entire place even became aware there had been an issue.

The chemotherapy was taking its toll, as well as its lumps of flesh out of Debbie. She was tired almost all the time. Although, the frequency and severity of the nauseousness did begin to alleviate as the program progressed, there never really was a time when

Debbie was completely in control of her own system. We continued to act as if nothing would ever go wrong, but we always knew that something could.

Debbie was also concurrently undergoing radiation treatment. The chemotherapy works in scatter shot fashion. Poison will find its way to the cancerous cells and will help to destroy them but has the setback that the poison will also destroy other parts of the body indiscriminately. Radiation attacks directly upon the location of the cancerous cells.

Debbie was placed on a stretcher like bed underneath a radiation machine that could direct small bursts of radiation energy where it was aimed. In Debbie's case it was aimed directly at the right front of her head. A firm mask of plastic gauze was created that fit precisely over Debbie's face and was then screwed down into the bed ensuring that Debbie could not move during the time the treatment was being administered. Debbie was obligated to lie completely still lest the radiation be directed to the undamaged and still healthy sections of her brain. This would have been calamitous. As remarked earlier, the passage of the radiation waves effectively burned out the roots of Debbie's hair, and although her hair did return to the rest of her head, it will never return to the right front quadrant.

We were never quite able to determine whether Debbie's side effects were solely the result of the chemotherapy or if they were the result of the radiation. There is a heightening effect to the symptoms of nausea when both therapies are used concurrently as they were in Debbie's case.

The months of dual chemotherapy and radiation treatments did indeed have their times of difficulty. The fact that Debbie, and I, survived them is a tribute to Debbie's steadfastness of purpose and to our ability to be flexible enough to accommodate whatever would be necessary to ensure Debbie's recovery. We maintained a schedule of walks that allowed us both to stay limber and maintain our respective muscle tones. I was fortunate because working for myself allowed us the ability to manipulate my work schedule to accommodate the increasing number of Debbie's doctor and radiation appointments.

The first of Debbie's follow-up and monitoring MRI's took place two months following her surgery. No tumor regrowth was observed at this time. Debbie was actively undergoing her chemotherapy and radiation treatments, getting outdoors to walk almost daily, and was clearly recovering from the trauma of her surgery. We began to think that the idea of Debbie returning back to work in the spring was not as outlandish as we might have first thought.

CHAPTER 17

Living with cancer, or any other life threatening disease, is like being on a roller coaster ride. You begin at the very bottom of a long hill and are completely unsure of how you got down there and additionally you are stuck with no earthly idea of how you will climb your way to the top of the slope that stands before you.

When we were faced with the reality of Debbie's diagnosis we really did not have many options. We could accept the advice of the doctors who had been assigned to us and had become our lifeline or we could refuse to accept treatment and stand idly by while the tumor ate out the insides of Debbie's brains. Like I said, we had few options.

There are some religious sects that will refuse the intervention of doctors and their modern medicines. Neither Debbie nor I belong to such a sect. We had no qualms about accepting the advice the physicians gave us. Debbie never wavered in her determination to get on with her life and to defeat this cancer that had literally brought her down shaking and quaking. We are certain we made the right decisions and we made following the orders of Debbie's doctors the number one priority of both of our lives.

Some people may receive advice from outside the field of medicine. Most notably many people recommended that we place our fate and Debbie's life in the hands of God. We appreciated the concern they expressed but Debbie's life, as well as yours and mine, are already in the hands of God. There is nothing more that we can do to elicit God's personal concern other than to ask him directly and in our own way.

Debbie was raised in a family of Methodists, I was raised a Jew. I did not insist we run to a synagogue and begin praying for relief utilizing the traditions of Judaism and neither did Debbie ask to be taken to a church to pray in a Methodist method. We both have a sincere belief that we do live in the presence of a higher power; we just don't believe that He lives in any single temple to the exclusion of others. I know that I did in my lonelier moments ask God for his help in caring for Debbie and although I can't necessarily say that He did any one particular thing to help us I can say that we were fortunate that Debbie lives in a time of miraculous medical advances and techniques that did not exist a few decades prior to Debbie's becoming ill. This fact alone has saved Debbie and if you wish to see the hand of God in this technological wave of advancement, then so be it. Certainly, I cannot deny it.

To all of the wonderful friends and family members who insisted we turn to Jesus, well we didn't. But, at the same time, we did. We just didn't give Him, She or It, that particular name.

We found the spirit of life in all of the things around us. Our short walks through the forest were suddenly more meaningful than all the hiking and traipsing about we had ever done before. There was symmetry to be found outdoors that emphasized our own existence. We were here and so were the trees, grasses, flowers, birds, insects, squirrels, foxes, and mountains. Suddenly we could see the difference between those things that are permanent, like the mountainside we trod upon, and those that are fleeting like the flowers that wilt in the fall, the insects that are eaten by others, and, well, us. We recognized that death is a part of the life cycle and that we would die and that dying would be part of the scheme of all things. The only determination we had was just to enjoy our time here together and to postpone that time of dying for as long as we could.

Debbie's first season as a brain cancer survivor progressed rapidly. There were always doctor appointments to keep, sessions of radiation to endure and our attempting to still be viable as a couple with a social agenda to keep our calendar filled. By the third month following her surgery it was clear that Debbie was still Debbie. The tumor and subsequent surgery had not stolen her personality.

We had successfully climbed that first hill that had stood before us and we began to make plans for Debbie's return to work. It would all depend upon the results of her next MRI that was scheduled for just after the beginning of the new year, 2002. We had Debbie take the scan and we went to visit Asheville once more to see the neurosurgeon. The doctor examined the latest pictures that been taken of the inside of Debbie's head and pronounced that she was tumor free at the present time. He stressed that this did not mean Debbie was cancer free. He explained that Debbie would never again be truly considered to be cancer free and that the tumor might reoccur at any time. He placed Debbie on a schedule of bi-monthly MRI's to monitor the tumor site and he also signed the waiver that would permit Debbie to begin driving and working again at the end of the six month waiting period for seizure patients as required by law.

We were ecstatic. This meant that Debbie could return to work on March 1st that coincidentally would have been her first day back at work following what in other years would have been her winter layoff.

The only medical issue that still required addressing was the question of Debbie's extreme weight loss. She was placed on a regimen of steroids to help her regain the weight and strength she had lost. She did, just like the baseball players of the nineties, bulk up. We laughed as to how she would no longer be able to play baseball or to take part in the Tour de France bicycle race. She was removed from the steroids after she had regained most but not all the weight she had lost due to chemotherapy. She was now actually quite svelte.

We decided to celebrate our reprieve from death by taking a trip off the mountain to a warmer and different locale. I had heard of the beauty of the Big Bend National Park located along the Mexican border in southwestern Texas. We decided to go there having done some research that told us that temperatures in February averaged near eighty degrees during the day. I called our friend Mike in Colorado and when I told him of our plans he said he would be able to join us for a week. We packed our car to the brim with camping gear and groceries and began our trip.

Debbie and I were on the road again and the fact of that alone was mind boggling and staggering to the imagination. Some might say miraculous- I won't argue.

We drove west stopping to see things we wanted and sometimes being amazed at what we saw. We took greater notice of the small towns we passed through stopping frequently to eat in small family owned restaurants where we were always pleasantly surprised by the goodness of the meals we were served. Debbie wore a baseball cap covering her head everywhere we went and no one was aware that just a few months before Debbie had endured major surgery.

One afternoon, a day's drive from our destination at Big Bend, we stopped at a state park called Monahans Sand Dunes. These were desert like dunes covering a several square mile area of the Great Plains. We parked at an overlook and began a short walk to the nearest peak of sand we could see. We arrived with no difficulty in fifteen minutes and set out a picnic and began to while away what was a drizzly afternoon. We began our return to the car and after awhile Debbie suggested that we might be walking in circles. I stopped and looked around and had the sudden realization that the entire landscape I could see in any direction looked exactly the same and I had no clue at all as to where we should go. I took a deep breath and decided to head for the highest dune we could see to reconnoiter. We approached and walked across our own footprints. We had returned to our picnic spot and I could see telephone poles about a half-mile off. Poles meant a road and we headed straight for the poles and we did find the road. Sheepishly we walked back down the road and located our car not soon after. We laughed and laughed in our gratefulness to be returned to civilization yet we remained determined to continue with our wilderness trip. Our flirt with disaster mirrored our fight against Debbie's tumor. We would ride with the tide and just keep swimming.

Our time spent in Big Bend was fantastic. It is a large land of prairie like desert with mountain ranges thrusting up from out of nowhere. The park is huge in size and there are various canyons to explore along the Rio Grande River as well as mountain ridges from which you can view the plains for hundreds of miles. We chose a remote wilderness campsite along the riverfront and in the instant I stepped from the car I was deafened by the silence that surrounded us. I had never heard the loudness of pure quiet before. It took me several minutes to adjust to it.

Our first night we were awakened by the sound of a large animal. It's call seemed remarkably loud as its "Hee-haw" echoed of the rock cliffs that bordered the narrow river on both sides. Debbie wondered what could be making such a racket and said she wished there was a ranger she could ask. I burst out and said in my best ranger voice imitation, "Why, that would be a donkey, ma'am." And from that day on, whenever one of us asked the other a stupid question, such as- "Would you like some coffee this morning?" Our answer would be, "Why, that would be a donkey, ma'am."

We explored a path that led along the ridge on the American side of the river and espying some steam rising up from the bamboos we went to investigate and discovered a hot spring. A primitive setting of rocks held the hot water in one place and after putting my hand in the water I determined that the temperature would be ideal for bathing. Over the next three weeks we would retire every evening to our hot spring and would soak for hours as the night stars would appear bringing with them the night's chill. The hot water would soak through to our bones heating our body core temperature to the point where we were comfortable enough standing naked in the cold night desert wind when we emerged to towel off and get dressed. We were still superheated as we returned to our campsite and would then cuddle together underneath the pile of sleeping bags, blankets and quilts we had brought along. Temperatures in the day would reach eighty but the night temperatures were fifty degrees lower and each morning we awoke to crustings of ice in our water containers. Debbie and I enjoyed the hot springs by ourselves a few nights and were thrilled to show our discovery to Mike when he arrived to join us.

One afternoon the three of us took an excursion across the river to a nearby Mexican village. We crossed the river on horseback and were guided by a local who promised to take care of us. I remember joking that someday I might write a book about our adventure and that the first line would be something similar to this one- "The bald woman led the way into the border town saloon followed by the two hairy gentlemen with parched tongues." I never wrote that book, but I'm glad I could slip that line in here.

We finished our Texas adventure with a visit to San Antonio and a look at the Alamo. We had dinner along the San Antonio Riverwalk before proceeding onto Austin where we saw Bob Dylan perform and then spent the night bar hopping in that music-loving city. We celebrated Debbie's birthday in a restaurant in Mississippi on Highway 61 and were home with a day to spare before Debbie and I had to return to work.

Our trip to Texas proved that Debbie could maintain a full days schedule of work and that she would not tire easily. The extended hiking we were doing was building up her strength quickly and we were ready to resume a more normal schedule of days.

We had conquered the first hill of our roller coaster ride, had stood at the top and enjoyed the "Wheeeee!" of our ride back down to the bottom. We just didn't know how long or how far we could get before we would have another mountain to face.

CHAPTER 18

Our life had changed drastically but if you were looking from the outside you may not have noticed any changes at all. Debbie was waking at 5:30 every weekday morning to be at work by seven. I was out of the house every day myself.

I had added a contract courier delivery service to my workload. Three days a week I delivered the water samples from various towns to be tested for impurities. I also picked up and delivered bank pouches and delivered them between the main office and the various bank branches. This required me to drive nearly 250 miles a day. This added contract on top of the landscape clients filled my workweek to its limit. I made sure that my weekends remained clear so that Debbie and I could have time together alone.

The chemotherapy program that Debbie had started was still underway. After the initial shocks to her system Debbie had begun to adjust rather well to the oral poisons she was ingesting. Incidents of nausea and vomiting had not disappeared altogether, but they had lessened. It was still possible at any moment for Debbie to begin to puke uncontrollably. It was no longer expected that she would do so. As I had mentioned earlier the oncologists had decided that Debbie would alternate between two different forms of chemotherapy. We could expect that there would be issues at the beginning of any new dosing regimen and we learned to stay at home on those days so that Debbie would have easier access to a commode. The weight loss the combination of radiation and chemotherapy were causing was still within reason and had not caused any undue concern yet.

After several months Debbie had completed her radiation treatments and her only medical appointments were the MRI's that were scheduled every two months. By the second or third one these had become routine. We had already begun the habit of going out for dinner when the MRI was complete and that is something we still do nearly ten years later.

We had also already become quite tired of the routine of repetitive paperwork we were forced to endure. At each MRI we were given a form in which we were to detail every medical procedure and surgery Debbie had ever been involved in. It was not acceptable to the office staff that Debbie had just filled out the same damn form two months before and that absolutely nothing except the date had changed. The first two times I went down the list with Debbie asking her about arthritis, heart disease, lung cancer, asthma, athlete's foot, etc. There was a list of at least sixty things, everything but hangnails. There was even a line asking if the patient had a penile implant. Debbie and I began checking "Yes" just to see what would happen and don't you know one day a nurse came out of the back room and asked about the penile implant. We explained that was just our private joke and that Debbie never had and probably never will have need for a penile implant. The nurse didn't think it was funny and made us begin a new form from scratch.

I also had time in that first year of Debbie's recovery to develop another pet peeve. It now seemed that almost all of our phone calls were coming from bill collection agencies. It reached the point where I began to be afraid every time the phone rang. This was incredibly aggravating in that it had been my desire to arrange satisfaction for the doctors and hospitals that cared for Debbie. I made sure they all had the correct insurance information and when the bills began to arrive for the portions of the bills not paid by insurance I arranged payment programs to satisfy the beast. Little did I know just how convoluted the process of hospital billing is.

For example, if Debbie had an MRI performed, Debbie would be billed by the hospital not once, but three separate times. Once by the hospital itself for the use of the MRI machine (usually about $3500-$4000), once for the injection of the dyes ($150-$200) used to give contrast to the scan and once for the radiologist ($400-$600) who reads the scan. I would receive the bill for the MRI and begin a payment program to the hospital. The hospital's accounting department would detract my payment from the one bill but then say that the other two were delinquent and would hire outside goons, called collection agencies, to hound us unmercifully. The fact that Debbie had been ordered to have an MRI every two months meant that within half a year we had many outstanding bills despite having had health insurance coverage and having instituted payment programs with our hospital.

One time a doctor ordered Debbie to undergo some blood work and Debbie proceeded to the lab where a technician drew a single vial of blood from her vein. It is bad enough that I am made queasy by the sight of blood; I still manage to stand by and hold Debbie's hand whenever I am allowed. What was really bad is that the one vial of blood created nineteen separate billing accounts in Debbie's name, one for each type of exam that the doctor had ordered.

I tried several times to deal with these people on the phone but they would not recognize that we had already cut our budget to the bone so that we could pay the bills we had incurred. I kept insisting that they treat Debbie as a single entity and bill her as one person. In other words, I asked that a single running total of Debbie's accounts be kept so that my payment to the hospital would satisfy all the artificially created separate accounts.

It's as if you went to the grocery and had to write separate checks or use separate credit cards to pay for each item. And the most important thing to remember is that you have a choice at the grocery not to purchase steak when you can only afford ground beef. At the hospital you are told what you must order and have no real option in shopping around. Can the families of the sick really afford to travel from town to town to price check hospitals? Even if this were a feasible thing to do, it would not matter as all hospitals charge about the same thing for all procedures. There maybe some regional discrepancies but basically the hospitals are charging as much as the insurance companies are willing to pay them. Neither the hospital nor insurance company administrator places the needs of the patient first. Their concern is the bottom line of an accounting ledger.

The story of Debbie would be incomplete if I didn't mention the financial disaster that a long-term health problem necessitates. The first thing that happens is that your insurance coverage rises. This rise will coincide with the necessity of missed work that the illness will require. Your insurance will eventually be transferred to the COBRA program. In the case of Debbie and I, her COBRA payment totaled over 90% of my take home pay. Unless you have the backing of several million dollars you can expect you will be unable to meet your expenses. I say several million because over the years I have been privy to the rates charged by hospitals for the use of their facilities. They are astronomical and beyond your imagination.

Again, lets use the example of the MRI machine. In 1996 I had a back operation and the orthopedic surgeon required I take an MRI to guide him in his surgery. I was billed nearly $3000 at that time and told the reason the cost was so high is because the hospital had just purchased the machine and needed to pay for it. Our hospital receives support from our county taxes, so in effect, the hospital used my money to buy the MRI, has been charging for its use for nearly fifteen years now and instead of lowering the price of scans (because surely the machine must be paid for by now) has raised the price of the scan nearly 33%.

Trust me when I say the hospitals will rip you off. They charged for every bandage used after Debbie's surgery and the cost of a band-aid would astonish you. Each individual tube she had been attached to was listed and I was appalled at the cost charged for plastic tubing. Debbie and I were using similar tubing in our beer making process and we would never have begun if I had to buy it at the price the hospital was charging for it. And don't whine about how the hospital stuff had to be sterile as so did the tubes we used to move beer from the brewing barrel to the bottles. There was a charge of $40 for a bar of soap.

I do not blame the doctors for this. Most doctors charge reasonable fees as compared to what the hospital will charge you for the use of its facilities. There are, of course, some doctors who are not worthy of their title who will charge for services they did not render or who will order unnecessary and duplicate tests just to pad their bills.

The bottom line is you can't afford a long-term illness yet you will be at the mercy of the health care institutions for the care you will need for yourself or your loved one.

I highly suggest that you go directly and in person to the finance office at your health care facility and insist that your payment program attach itself to all accounts that may be created in your name. I also recommend seeking legal advice to help you deal with unwanted bill collectors.

You will always be better off dealing directly with the hospital than with a collection agency. First off a collection agency will accept half of your payment as their fee- the hospital will never see that cash. Secondly, it is your right not to be hassled in your home or at your place of employment by a bill-collecting agency. Insist upon that right! You may have to place that request in writing- do it. The peace of mind you will have at home demands it. The quiet your convalescing loved one will have demands it.

Don't ever feel guilty or badly that you are leaving bills half settled. To begin with the hospital is doing quite well on the 80 or 90 percent of your bill that your insurance company has already paid them. Being honest, as I have tried to be, your payment program of whatever you can actually afford without cutting back on necessities like food and heat, will be sufficient enough for the hospital administrators to travel to conventions in tropical locales. For your own well-being try to not be so bitter about the game, just play it.

Let me explain this way. The hospital knows you are a dreadfully ill person who will require their care for the rest of your lifetime. They also know you will lose any private insurance you may have within a short time. They recognize if you are a Medicare patient already and know when you can become certified as one. They also know that Medicare requires its beneficiaries to curb back their savings to a recognized amount. They also know that your policy (private or otherwise) will only pay 80% of your bill. Therefore the finance office knows that in order to get the most for their services they charge as much as the government will allow. This doesn't mean they didn't do a great job and save your life. It just means they will overcharge purposely to get back as much as they can. They do this by performing every test imaginable and charging insane amounts like the aforementioned $40 bar of soap.

Now all of this costs us as a society in some way. The legitimate bills and expenses must be paid for. We could all assume a fair share by paying a premium to an impartial non-profit agency, such as our government. That would also create the largest possible risk group and would save us all in two ways. First our premiums would be less because of the lower risk group. Second, the profit motive would be taken out of the entire system. All we have supported is insurance company executives and the bankers who gamble on them. None of this money is going to make the hospitals better. Nurses and technicians are not getting raises. In fact, they are being asked to work longer shifts for less pay, endangering the safety of every patient. And yes, it would require the wealthy in our country to pay their fair share.

And what is that fair share? OK, there's room for haggling there. The recent fight over the rescinding of the Bush tax cut is an example. People who earned a million dollars or more a year were asked to pay an additional 2% of their yearly income. That's $20,000. But it's also out of a million, also known as $1,000,000, for God sakes! I wasn't even taking home but a few thousand a year and I was still paying my taxes and Debbie's inflated insurance premiums.

Remember the story of the lady who complained I couldn't mow her lawn because I was caught up in the hospital as Debbie had an emergency craniotomy. She was a millionaire many times over. Her summer home, that I helped maintain, sold for well over $6 million dollars. She only lived there two months a year. I never begrudged any of that to her but I must say her priorities were a tinge warped when she equated my missing a landscape appointment to Debbie's brain surgery. This is the same deal. The $20,000 the millionaires pay in taxes keeps people alive. It finds jobs for those who need them. The only difference it makes now is the difference between a $400 dollar bottle of wine and a $200 dollar bottle twice a week! We're not even talking about people who have accumulated a million dollars- just ones who earn that much in a single year. Oh, and I know that everyone has worked for their wealth. Debbie and I always worked too. We don't ask for the buying power to drink the expensive wine but we do say unequivocally that our life is worth as much as anybody's, wealthy millionaire or not.

I have always from the beginning of her illness sheltered Debbie from this side of our life. We shared a checking account prior to her illness; Debbie also had her own account for her personal use like buying gifts for her husband. I have never discussed the charges and fees that her illness has created. They are not her fault and they are not her concern. Her concern is staying alive and as healthy as possible and that is enough for her to deal with.

On our sixth wedding anniversary and the first anniversary of Debbie's surgery we took a week off from work and flew out to Colorado to visit our friends Mike and Debbie and to join with them at a concert being held at the Red Rocks Amphitheater outside of Denver. This was an incredible milestone for the two of us. It was truly a blessing that Debbie had survived this year. Many brain tumor patients do not.

We spent several marvelous days seeing the Rocky Mountains utilizing Mike's four-wheel drive vehicle. We were able to witness tremendous canyons and mountain ridges from little traveled back roads. One day we started down a steep canyon and emerged into the wilderness of the Colorado Sand Dunes. We spent nearly thirty minutes just to climb to the edge of a single dune. We traversed the high country of the Rocky Mountain National Park and completed the adventure by enjoying a performance by Robert Plant of Led Zeppelin fame in Denver the night before our return flight home.

So, life went on at our house in the mountains. Change had occurred but it was underneath the surface. I had become callous in my dealing with certain people and agencies and had no tolerance with those who did not respect our right to privacy in our home. This callousness has changed who I am. The brain surgery had not changed Debbie's personality; it had changed mine.

Debbie and I continued our love for each other. We still slept together joyfully and found comfort in each other's presence. Our weekends were still spent in glorious walks through the mountain trails. By the end of the first year after Debbie's surgery and the six clean MRI reports we had received we began to not dread the appointments as much. We just assumed everything was fine and would continue that way.

The life of a cancer patient is never serene, however, and the next cycle of our roller coaster ride was about to begin.

CHAPTER 19

By the early spring of 2003, almost a year and a half following Debbie's surgery a shadow emerged on Debbie's latest MRI. The oncologists agreed this was the beginning of the regrowth of the cancerous tumor.

Three different doctors were seeing Debbie at this time. We were still making trips bi-monthly to visit with Dr. Rhoton who you will remember was the neurosurgeon who did the original surgery. Debbie was also being seen by Dr. Gray, a medical oncologist who was affiliated with our local hospital, and by Dr. Mack, a radiation oncologist who was also located locally. These three doctors conferred via telephone and internet and their treatment decisions were made collectively.

Dr. Mack, an attractive and petite woman, also took care to make sure that the rest of Debbie's health issues would not go uncared for. As a matter of course Dr. Mack added general practitioner to the list of chores she took responsibility for. She also designed and implemented the radiation therapy program that Debbie had undergone. Both Debbie and I enjoyed our dealings with Dr. Mack. She was clearly devoted to the overall well being of her patients and her buoyant attitude made visits to her office a pleasant experience. She would encourage Debbie to utilize her sense of humor and she seemed to have an authentic liking for us as a couple.

Dr. Gray, was a young man for a doctor, probably still in his thirties. It became his responsibility to determine the types of chemotherapy Debbie would be forced to endure and then to administer them effectively. It was Dr. Gray who stood up to the insurance company when they at first refused to pay for Debbie's prescribed chemotherapy pills.

Debbie and I believed we had the best care available and were happy with the way we were treated. We had already seen how the doctors would be honest with us and would tell us point blank that they needed to do more research upon certain things. The chemotherapy regimen was certainly a case in point.

Brain cancer patients are relatively rare equaling only 2% of all the cancer patients in the United States. Drs. Gray and Mack had relatively little experience with a brain tumor patient. They spent much of their time researching Debbie's illness and conferring through the use of the internet with other specialists throughout the country concerning best treatment options. They had earned our trust and we respected their opinions. We had been warned that Debbie's tumor was cancerous and might reoccur. We were not shocked and we waited to see what option of treatment the doctors would arrive with.

Basically, there were three choices. The first would be to do a second craniotomy and to physically remove the reemerging tumor. This was decided against as it was felt the surgery would still leave over the microscopic bits of tumor that a scalpel could not reach. Secondly, Debbie could be dosed with another round of chemotherapy and thirdly, Debbie could receive more radiation.

A new technology had developed. This was called stereotactic radiosurgery and involved a most precise method of blasting mega doses of radiation directly upon the affected site inside Debbie's brain. Although similar to the radiation therapy Debbie had already undergone it differed in the strength of the individual beams that would be shot into Debbie's head. The radiation regimen involved many treatments of smaller dosages of radiation in the hope that the accumulation of "rads" would destroy the tumor. The stereotactic radiosurgery procedure would blast tremendous amounts of energy at the tumor site attempting to destroy it in one fell swoop.

It was never said or thought that the original treatments of radiation and chemotherapy had failed to do their job. They had. Debbie had successfully survived the first year of her cancer and that is the year that proves statistically to be fatal to many brain cancer patients. Debbie's overall health and strength at the time of her presentation played a large factor in her quick recovery from surgery. The nature of her tumor to not metastasize also contributed to her survival.

Debbie, in the meanwhile, was not suffering effects from the new tumor growth. It was still so small in size that it was felt the doctors had enough time to do the research and still be able to effectively treat the regrowth. She was still maintaining her full work schedule and was in the midst of her spring cleanup and planting. She was busy at work and maintained her work schedule only missing days when she was required to be at a doctor's appointment.

When the doctors agreed that the new method of stereotactic radiosurgery was the best bet in their opinion to treat the tumor we had no objection to going along with them and arrangements were made through Dr. Rhoton's office to have the procedure done in Asheville. It was here that trouble began to arise and I am convinced that payment issues played a factor.

The radiologist Dr. Rhoton had introduced us to had met with us and explained the procedure to us. We set a date for the administration of the treatment and shuffled our work schedules to allow us to be able to attend. The evening before the scheduled operation we received a call from the hospital telling us their equipment was in need of repair and we were asked if we would be able to reschedule for two weeks later. I was quite willing to accommodate and rescheduled. The next two months saw the procedure cancelled and rescheduled three or four times. Each time we received some lame excuse as to why it couldn't be performed and each time I rescheduled the procedure. After a few months of this cat and mouse game I began to be concerned that in the meantime the tumor was growing unchecked in Debbie's head and must be dealt with. I arranged through Dr. Mack to have the procedure done at a hospital in Charlotte and it was performed there in July.

Although I will never know for sure I believe that the insurance company had refused to pay the Asheville hospital for what was at the time a new and innovative treatment.

Instead of being honest with me and telling me this they continued to postpone Debbie's treatment in hopes they would be able to administratively clear the way for the payment that the insurance company never had a moral right to refuse in the first place. This postponement was dangerous and was threatening Debbie's health. The Charlotte program had been able to work its way through the red tape bureaucracy and scheduled and completed the treatment.

Following this debacle Debbie and I ended our relationship with Dr. Rhoton and with the hospital in Asheville. We will always be thankful for the expertise and skill of Dr. Rhoton. It was his initial proficiency that allowed Debbie to survive her brain surgery. I am still, nearly ten years later, making a monthly payment to Dr. Rhoton's office to satisfy the bill we incurred with his office. I don't believe he is still affiliated with that office but it is a debt of honor that we continue to acknowledge.

The treatment itself involved Debbie being placed in a room the size of an indoor handball court with a planetarium like projector hanging from the ceiling. Debbie would be placed in the middle of the room and the maximum amount of "rads" a human could endure would be directed precisely unto the tumor site. To facilitate this Debbie was forced to have a halo screwed into her head that would guide the radiologist in his aiming of the rays. The doctor had prescribed a single pill of valium for Debbie to ingest prior to the procedure. We protested that this would be insufficient and we turned out to be right. Debbie suffered severe discomfort and some pain during the operation.

After doing the doctor's office shuffle where we waited patiently in a back room the doctor finally arrived with a Sears toolbox in hand. He injected painkiller into four sites surrounding Debbie's head and I instantly was able to see large swelling at the injection sites. He then opened the toolbox from which he removed a common screwdriver. He literally screwed four distinct screws into Debbie's head directly into the swollen areas and mounted the halo onto Debbie's head. It was truly grotesque, a cross between a football helmet and a pair of goggles with a white plastic visor. The doctor asked Debbie to be sure that the toolbox containing the screwdriver was transported with her wherever she might be taken to ensure that the halo could be removed quickly in case of emergency. I sat with Debbie while she waited for the operation to begin. She was in some discomfort and I was helpless to assist her. Finally she was wheeled out for a pre-surgery MRI with the halo on her head and then the treatment itself was administered.

After an hour spent in a step down room Debbie was released. The entire thing from arrival to departure had taken about half a day. Debbie was feeling well and so we took advantage of the day and traveled on to Asheville where we joined some friends at the Bele Chere outdoor music festival. Debbie was remarkable. No one could have conceived that she had been screwed four times over just that morning.

CHAPTER 20

We have added a new game to our daily routine. We are now using hand signals and are trying to substitute them instead of the meaningless phrases that Debbie has used for the last two years.

Debbie's personality has become hidden so deep under the monotone voice that she has adopted that it is almost impossible for me to determine just what it is she means when she speaks. She mumbles constantly and I must frequently ask her to speak up even though I am aware that most likely all she has said is one of the four stock phrases that she uses to discuss everything. "Yeah", "right", "good" and "OK" are used to discuss the news, the weather, the program on the TV, the birds at our feeders, just everything. Debbie, although still capable, has developed this awful habit of just neglecting to speak in coherent sentences.

I have tried everything to engage her in deeper conversations and to make her aware of her monosyllabic responses to everything. Debbie will sit down in her chair and say, "Yeah." I'll repeat "yeah" and exaggerate the rise in my voice to help ensure that Debbie recognizes the question form. Debbie will once again repeat in the monotone, "Yeah". We will repeat this word "yeah" back and forth several times until Debbie finally realizes that I am asking for some elucidation on her part and she will look at me triumphantly and state in that monotone I have come to abhor, "Right." I will inquire as to what is right and Debbie may say "she doesn't know" or "nothing". I will exclaim in surprise, "Nothing's right?" and she will respond monotonously, "Right." As you can deduce the level of our intellectuality does leave a little something to be desired.

I am determined to pierce Debbie's shell and to get her to laugh and smile. Sometimes she will go into series mode and combine her "yeah, right and good" into a single outburst. "The holy trinity", I holler. "My baby says yeah, right and good!" I sing aloud to whatever melody crosses my mind at the time. Debbie sometimes grins. She knows that I am teasing her out of love but that does not mean that she necessarily enjoys being teased. She just doesn't really see that her speech has degenerated to these grunts of meaningless sounds.

Debbie does sometimes encourage herself by whispering "yeah" repeatedly to herself. As she struggles to walk to the bathroom, or to rise up from her easy chair she will intone countless numbers of "yeahs" as if she is a cheerleader imploring her team to score. She is so engaged in the physical activity of movement that she is totally unaware that she has repetitively mumbled "yeah" aloud thirty times or more.

I have attempted to actually count the frequency with which Debbie will use the word "yeah" in a day. I began on one of those days that Debbie did not arise before noon and I felt obligated to stir her from her bed at one in the afternoon so that she could have some breakfast. She had said "yeah" over thirty times before she had even made it to the commode. There were eighty "yeahs" by the time she finished dressing and another twenty to walk from her bedroom to her easy chair where I presented her with a cup of coffee. Her response upon accepting the cup, you guessed it- "yeah". By the time my count had reached over 200 "yeahs" Debbie had been barely awake a single hour and I could not go on counting. I estimate I listen to a few thousand "yeahs" a day give or take a hundred or so.

My wife has clearly become slower in her mental processes as well as in her physical attributes. She hears things but does not understand what she has heard until a few moments have passed. This is thoroughly disconcerting to me and sometimes dangerous to her. There have been several instances where Debbie begins to do something such as reaching into a corner of the room to retrieve something she has dropped. Debbie has difficulty in maneuvering herself and maintaining her balance when she is placed in tight spaces and corners, by definition, are tight spaces. I call out and ask her to stop, but she continues, and often the result is a crashing fall to the ground. I lift her, of course, and then ask if she didn't hear me say, "Stop!" She says she did so I press forward and ask her why she didn't just stop. The answer is invariably, "I don't know." And she doesn't know. The hearing of the command and the processing and understanding of the command just do not happen in synchronicity.

I do so want Debbie to understand that I am here to keep her safe and that I love and care for her. I recognize these cognitive issues and want her to smile through them so, I have begun to act out her phrases for her.

"Yeahs" have become two thumbs up.

"Right" is now the raising of the left arm at a ninety-degree angle from the elbow as if I was a driver signaling a right turn.

"Good" is the signal of a football referee signifying touchdown or the success of a field goal attempt.

Debbie says, "Yeah" and I give her two thumbs up. "Good" she continues, and my arms fly upwards to the sky. This bit of idiocy on my part has intrigued Debbie and she has begun repeating my motions. She has joined in the game and this actually is good! I have caused her to smile and become engaged in something outside herself and as an extra added bonus have gotten her to indulge in a tiny bit of movement and exercise.

Good!

CHAPTER 21

Following Debbie's endurance of the stereotactic radiosurgery procedure we returned to our normal routine of work and then weekend relaxation. All appeared to be in tip-top shape and the first several MRI's that were taken after the procedure showed no substantial changes taking place inside Debbie's brain. Debbie was still vibrant and strong and had no difficulty in returning back to her full-time position. She was still receiving health insurance issued by her employer but the rates had risen for her and her take home pay was significantly affected. I was continuing to work both my landscaping and courier jobs and we were continuing to meet our financial obligations. In fact, we had been doubling and tripling up on our mortgage payments for so long that we had come near to paying off our house. I continued to shunt as much cash as possible toward our mortgage. I wasn't sure why at the time but a few years later I understood that action might have been the very best financial thing I had ever done.

Over the years I had done some pretty dumb things too. Most notably I had sold the house I had been living in when I left to go to Georgia and teach school. When I returned three years later the housing market had already doubled and I was unable to purchase a home with the square footage that I had once enjoyed. I did buy a reconverted trailer and it is here that we still live today. We have, as previously stated, added onto our trailer base. To my way of thinking that promotes us from plain white trash to upscale white trash with all the rights and privileges that entails.

We now needed to replace Dr. Rhoton in our pantheon of medical experts. Dr. Gray had also moved on to another position and although Dr. Godwin, a kind, elderly gentleman had adequately replaced him, we really had no more use for a medical oncologist as Debbie had completed her chemotherapy. Dr. Mack continued to see Debbie as a general practitioner ensuring Debbie's other health needs were attended to; but Debbie had also completed the radiation program. In fact, with the mega dose of radiation Debbie had just received through stereotactic radiosurgery we were informed that Debbie would never be allowed to undergo any radiation again.

Drs. Mack, Godwin and Gray had already been utilizing the resources of the Brain Tumor Center at Duke University to do much of their research and an inquiry was made to see if they would accept Debbie as a patient. An appointment was arranged and we traveled to Durham where the university is located.

We met with Dr. Henry Friedman who is the director of the Brain Tumor Clinic. He is a jovial person and upon seeing Debbie and I waiting in his examination room he asked boisterously, "Haven't I seen you at the Fillmore East?" Now the Fillmore East was a concert venue managed by Bill Graham in New York City back in the sixties. It closed its operations in 1971 and the craziest thing about Dr. Friedman's question is that he very well may have seen me back then. I was fortunate enough to have attended a few shows there back in the day when I was still riding the subway into Manhattan as a teenager. I will never know how Dr. Friedman was able to so accurately identify me as a New Yorker or how he could peg either Debbie or I as a "deadhead". We were both long past the stage of wearing tie-dye t-shirts in public.

We had already been aware of Duke's reputation as being in the forefront of care for patients with brain tumors. Patients travel from around the country to be treated there. (Senator Edward Kennedy chose Duke as his facility of care when he was faced with his tumor a few years later.) Dr. Friedman detailed the advantages that Debbie would have being treated there and we began what to this day has continued as a beneficial experience for Debbie.

Dr. Friedman did say one thing that disturbed us. He stated that he would not have chosen the stereotactic radiosurgery as the means to treat Debbie's tumor recurrence. His choice would have been a second bout of chemotherapy cocktails. His words were prescient.

I do recall one of Debbie's first clinic appointments at Duke. A young male resident was administering some neurological exams to Debbie. Touch your thumb to each of your fingers as quickly as you can, lift all limbs on command, follow the path of my penlight by just moving your eyes and things like that. At one point he said that Debbie should stand with her arms stretched out and then to reach with her index finger and touch my nose. Debbie did exactly that. The doctor jumped back sputtering that she should touch her nose, not his. Debbie had followed his literal command.

The exam continued and the resident asked Debbie to solve some simple math equations. Now arithmetic was never Debbie's strongest suit even in the best of times. She did all right with the 2+2=4 stuff but when the problems became more advanced Debbie began to take more time before giving her solutions. The one that stumped her was 106-38. Debbie was trying her best. I'm not positive she could ever have solved that without a calculator and as the minutes passed the doctor said that would be sufficient. He made a notation in the chart and went down the corridor to his next appointment. More than ten minutes had passed as we waited patiently for the next doctor to examine Debbie when she suddenly jumped up from the examining table and ran into the hallway calling out as loud as she could, "Sixty-eight, sixty-eight!" Debbie was correct, 106-38=68. She was just ten minutes too late.

Soon after starting with Duke we were introduced to a young resident named Annick Desjardins. Dr. Desjardins had grown up in Montreal and has a delightful French accent that seems to emphasize her vibrant and bubbly personality. Over the years she has become Debbie's doctor of record and has performed over and beyond the call of service. We will be forever grateful for her kindness and her expertise.

Having arranged our medical ducks in a row Debbie and I proceeded to schedule for another cross-country trip to take place during the winter season of January and February but first we were called to New York to help bury my father.

George passed away on September 16, 2003. He had been suffering the later stages of Alzheimer's disease and had been confined to a nursing home for the last three years. Debbie had only had the opportunity to meet him a few times before his deterioration. She had always adored his sense of humor and particularly enjoyed the way he would entertain us in restaurants by taking the linen napkins and folding them in such a way that when unfolded the napkin would resemble a brassiere. Debbie could instantly see from where my own raunchy sense of humor had been born. My dad's death was not an unexpected one, he was 81 years young when he died, but it was a sad time for those who knew him. He had always been the life of any gathering he was part of as he had demonstrated at our wedding by sharing his "baby picture". He had taught me how to be responsible when I was still just a child. I never forgot the lessons he taught that a man should be judged by his actions.

My dad's last years were unfortunate. He was unable to communicate and could no longer remember my face the last time I saw him. We would visit him and take him outdoors for a walk. He would bend over and pick up a rock or shell and examine it for hours. Sometimes I catch Debbie doing something similar and I cringe inside.

As my father had requested the funeral was held in accordance with the strictest rules of Jewish orthodoxy. Debbie was being introduced to many of my cousins for the very first time and was a bit nervous about not doing anything to offend anyone. I assured her she should not worry, as I was proud to introduce her to all. I had the pleasure of introducing Debbie to Rabbi Solomon, my Hebrew School teacher when I was a boy studying for my Bar Mitzvah. He recognized immediately that Debbie was suffering some illness or other and wished her good health. My mother informed me later that week that the Rabbi had lost his wife to cancer just a short while before. I wish I had known that so that I would have been able to console him as he was consoling us.

At the conclusion of the service we each took turns with a shovel spilling a spadeful of dirt unto my father's casket. After each had taken a turn Debbie and I seized the two tools provided and completed the task of covering my father's grave. I will never forget the scene of Debbie, just two years after her own brain surgery and dressed formally in a black dress, using her landscape skills to help me bury my dad while many younger and healthier people stood by and wondered who she was. A mitzvah is a good deed. Debbie did a mitzvah that afternoon and continued to perform good deeds for the rest of the week as she sat the seven day "shiva" mourning period required by orthodox Jews. Debbie's full acceptance into my family was assured by the end of that week of memories and reminiscences.

We chose the southwest for our winter getaway and traveled to Tucson where my nephew Adam had moved. We explored the Saguaro National Park and were enthralled with the tall stately cactus. This was the first exposure Debbie or I had experienced in the deep southwest and we enjoyed it. We spent a couple of nights across the California border in Joshua Tree National Park before leaving our camping behind and going decadently to a hotel suite in San Diego. We spent several drizzly days in San Diego walking along the beaches that featured towering cliffs overlooking the ocean and another day in the rain at the San Diego Zoo. We loved our time in San Diego but we joked about how the Chamber of Commerce had lied to us. We discovered that it does rain in southern California!

We returned home in time to begin the spring season of 2004 feeling refreshed and hoping that there would be no health issues for us to deal with in the upcoming year.

CHAPTER 22

The spring and summer went as smoothly as any year since the onset of Debbie's cancer. Debbie maintained her schedule of bi-monthly MRI scans and we returned to Duke every four months for a personal examination by the doctors there. A routine developed in which we would arrive at Duke with the films of her latest MRI and would receive the report as to what the doctors saw on them. On the months we did not report personally to Duke the films were mailed to Duke and the doctor would call us at home with her reading. I was also examining the films as they were in my possession from the time they were taken at our local hospital until I hand delivered them to the receptionist at the Brain Tumor Clinic in Durham. The films clearly showed the section of Debbie's brain that had been operated upon and the key was to look very closely at the borders of that area to see if anything new or different was present. I began to become quite adept at reading Debbie's MRI and Dr. Desjardins jokingly called me Dr. Block, junior radiologist.

At one visit early in the fall I pointed to a white cloudy area on the film and mentioned that this should receive closer examination. Our serenity was once more shattered. Dr. Desjardins took the films into another room to confer with her colleagues and they all agreed that what I had noticed was probably scar tissue or necrosis that had been caused by the radiation Debbie had received.

At the next MRI the section of necrotic tissue had grown. It was explained that the radiation had caused some of the capillary blood vessels in Debbie's brain to burst and that the necrosis was the clotted remains of the blood. It was decided that the one and only sure way to identify the nature of this new type of growth inside Debbie was to have her undergo a brain biopsy. The MRI, although an amazing tool, does not present an actual photograph of the inside of your body, just a graphic representation and without an actual microscopic examination of tissue it is impossible to identify the unknown tissue with total accuracy.

Before the doctors would perform the biopsy, however, it was determined that one other diagnostic tool should be utilized. This is the PET scan. PET stands for Positron Emissions Tomography. Tomography is a fancy word for mapping. Positrons are radioactive particles. An injection of radioactive sugar is given and the theory is that because cancer cells are the fastest growing cells in your body the doctors would be able to determine the rate in which the sugar is ingested. The scanner itself is remarkably similar to the MRI so there was no real difference to Debbie in the form of scan performed. The only difference I could see was in the injection itself. When the radioactive sugar was injected I could follow it as it worked its way up the vein of Debbie's arm. It appeared as a silvery lump inside Debbie's vein. It was quite weird looking but did not cause any undue discomfort to Debbie. If there were cancer cells present they would appear on the PET scan since they would be "eating" the sugar the fastest.

After both the MRI and PET were found to be inconclusive it was determined to go forward with the biopsy to discover exactly what it was that was going on inside Debbie's head.

We arrived in mid-December at the Duke University Hospital for the biopsy to be performed. We laughed at the acronym the hospital employees wore on their nametags. DUH- Duke University Hospital. We had prepared for this and Debbie was wearing the baseball cap a friend had given her. The cap featured a cartoon of an intoxicated person with a sickly grin pointing to their head and saying "Duh". Debbie received smiles and giggles from every nurse, aide, technician and doctor who saw her cap. Several asked if they could purchase it.

We were rooting for necrosis and against the reoccurrence of tumorous matter. The biopsy was a miniature version of the craniotomy Debbie had undergone three years before. In this case, a small needle like hole was made in Debbie's skull and a tiny probe was introduced to swab the area that needed further identification. The material removed would be examined in minute detail by a pathologist who would then be able to make a determination of what it was. Unfortunately for Debbie a halo needed to be once again screwed into her head to guide the neurosurgeon in his placing of the needle and the swab. Once more she was forced to endure screws being placed in her skull and to wear the unwieldy helmet device until the completion of the operation. I do not know from what wellspring of courage and bravery Debbie has been able to draw from in order to endure these indignities on her body. She just does and I have always been in awe of her calm. The morning of this biopsy, however, was one of the few times I have seen her in tears.

The neurosurgeon arrived in our hospital room before six in the morning to screw the halo in place. Debbie's surgery was scheduled second that morning and the painkillers Debbie had been given began to wear off before the operation had begun. She began to complain of severe pain from the screws inserted in her head and the nurses could do nothing because the neurosurgeon who must give the orders for more painkillers was still involved in his first surgery of the day and could not be reached. The extra hour of enforced waiting was hell for Debbie, for the nurse who tried to comfort her and for me who was helpless once more to do anything other than hold her hand. Thankfully remembrances of pain do not last and Debbie has forgotten most of that morning. And thankfully Debbie was finally brought to the operating room, the biopsy was performed, and by the end of the afternoon we had received the good news that Debbie's pathology report stated that the tumor was not present at this time and the mass now developing in her head was nothing but necrotic tissue.

An interesting coincidence took place that afternoon as Debbie recovered in her room following the procedure. Along with the endless stream of doctors and nurses who came to continuously check on Debbie's condition we received a visit from an elderly woman who introduced herself as Pastor Friedman. The pastor asked if we would like to speak with her concerning spiritual matters and Debbie declined her invitation. Before she left our room, however, my curiosity overcame me and I asked Pastor Friedman what denomination she represented. To my mind Friedman was just not a common name for a pastor. I was right, of course, and Pastor Friedman explained that she was a rabbi and that she introduced herself as a pastor so as not to frighten the overwhelming majority of non-Jews who were patients in the hospital. She went on to explain that she had noticed the name Block on the patient list and had made a special trip to visit with us. She elaborated that when she was a young child growing up in Brooklyn she had attended a Hebrew school where she was taught by a Rabbi Block. She remembered that he was not only her teacher (the Hebrew word rabbi means teacher) but that he was also the principal of the school and his first name was Chaim. I was stunned but I was also pleased then to introduce myself and to tell her that Chaim had been my grandfather. We talked and she reminisced about her childhood in Brooklyn for half an hour before she continued her rounds bringing comfort to the sick. Quite a coincidence and only in Durham, I thought. When I related this story to my mother she was as delighted as I had been with the proof once more that we live in a very small world indeed and that we are all interconnected.

Debbie and I returned home with another start. Tumors were not growing, she was still cancer free as the holiday season approached and we prepared to make a visit to see Debbie's mom and to enjoy Christmas with her. Debbie had no issues to deal with, but I did.

I had lost my job as a courier. On the day following the presidential election of 2004 I went into one of the bank branches I had been delivering to and one of the tellers who I had been conversing with for over a year asked me if it wasn't such a great thing that President Bush had been reelected and didn't his election represent a victory for moral Americans. I honestly responded, "Sure it did if you believe that morality includes bombing and making war on innocent civilians, women and children." The teller exploded in a violent rage and demanded to know how could I possibly say such a thing. When I answered her by saying, "Because it's the truth" she exploded anew. I continued to finish my route for the day but the teller had complained to the fellow I was contracting from that I had created a scene at the bank. This placed my employer in a delicate position and he felt obligated to release me. I had done nothing wrong other than to calmly express my opinion in response to a direct question but I was let go.

That evening I wrote a short letter to my friends explaining what had happened and asking them to remove any bank accounts they might have as a protest against my dismissal and sent it via e-mail. For the next month I became a celebrity of sorts and discovered what it is like to have your fifteen minutes of fame. It is overrated.

What happened was that some of my friends were so incensed by my story that they reproduced my letter and sent it to their friends who then reproduced my letter and sent it to their friends who then reproduced my letter and sent it to their friends who then....well, you get the idea. By the end of the week I had been contacted by several newspapers and by National Public Radio. I was interviewed on NPR via a phone link and I began receiving hundreds of e-mails from people all around the country who thanked me for speaking my mind and wished me success in my future. It was quite a whirlwind for a while and it was gratifying to know I was not alone. I was interviewed in my home by a reporter/photographer from the Charlotte Observer who used my predicament to reinforce the falsehood that it was I who had created a disturbance. You would have thought that a newspaper would back the usage of free speech and the exchange of ideas but you would be wrong.

The bank itself did have a public relations nightmare on their hands and I was told that they had to have several operators on hand to answer calls concerning the dismissal of messenger Jeff Block. I had no qualms about having caused this disturbance in their routine as no one from the bank cared enough to ever contact me and ask my side of the story which was basically that I had just responded honestly and calmly to a direct question that had been placed to me.

I was glad for the moral support but what I needed was a job and I was able to find one before we took off to Florida. I was hired as a teacher at a nearby residential facility which housed and cared for children who had been adjudicated by a court as a sex offender. These children were of all ages from six to seventeen and were of both sexes. Since I had an elementary school license to teach I was designated as the teacher for those students in grades K-6. The reality was that I dealt with students across all the grade levels since the classes were assigned with the psychological needs of the children as the first priority with disregard for actual age or grade level. This is the last job I have held and I maintained it until Debbie's ever worsening condition required me to stay at home and care for Debbie on a full time basis.

We spent Christmas in Florida with Debbie's mom but we were unable to take an extended winter vacation that year, as I now had to return and begin my duties as a schoolteacher.

CHAPTER 23

Debbie began the new year of 2005 looking great and feeling strong. The scans and biopsy of late December showed that the only happening taking place inside Debbie's brain was the growing mass of necrotic or dead tissue. No tumor was present at this time and Debbie was looking forward to beginning back at work when March and spring cleanup began again. The cycle of Debbie's year was complete and she spent much time at home preparing flowerbed designs for the upcoming season. She began work with no idea that this would be the last year she would ever work.

When the necrosis had first began to appear on scans the previous fall Debbie had been placed once again on steroids. The purpose this time was not to help Debbie gain weight but to help prevent the bleeding inside her brain that was causing the buildup of the necrotic tissue. Of course, Debbie did begin to gain weight and ballooned clear up to 200 pounds. Debbie would be taken off the steroids and her weight would settle back down, but then it was back on the steroids as the internal brain bleeding is life threatening and a little extra weight is not. This up and down of weight gain and loss became Debbie's own little personal roller coaster within the larger roller coaster we both faced as we continued determinedly to not allow Debbie's illness to change our lives anymore than necessary.

For the first time in several years I did not have the flexibility with my work schedule as I had enjoyed. Fortunately my weekends were free and even though I did attend some Saturdays to give extra support to my students at some extra-curricular event or other for the most part the weekends were time for Debbie and I to do things together.

I thought little of it at the time but Debbie began to beg off from some of the weekend walks I wished her to take with me. I was disappointed and felt neglected but I made no connection to her sometimes refusals and her brain issues. I should have.

Debbie still accompanied me frequently and showed no physical signs of debilitation as spring advanced towards summer.

We had spoken over the years of traveling through the desert and red rock canyons of southeast Utah. I had been there many years ago and wanted to share the beauty and spirit of this part of the country with Debbie. My new job was to allow me a three-week hiatus at the beginning of July and I began to lobby Debbie to request some time off and join me in a trip out west. This was not an easy thing for Debbie to ask. Summer is the height of her landscaping season but she was able to convince her boss that her assistant could handle things in her absence and it was compromised that Debbie could use her accrued holiday time to take a week. This combined with the 4th of July weekend gave her a window of ten days free and it was agreed that I would drive out west alone and pick Debbie up at the airport in Salt Lake City.

I left as soon as I was released from my last day of class and enjoyed the freedom of my independent cross-country drive. I met with my nephew Adam and spent a night camping with him in the backcountry of Arizona's Petrified Forest. That was a wonderful experience and we were witness to a rarity- the blooming of a moonflower. I awoke early that morning and climbed the nearest ridge and became one with the landscape as the sun rose and colored each of the rocks and ridges of the Painted Desert in gentle pastels.

Adam and I continued together to Canyon de Chelly in northeastern Arizona and stood in awe of the sheer cliffs towering 800-1000 feet over the canyon floor. We were privileged to make the acquaintance of a Navajo Indian who lived there. He befriended us and gifted us with a horseback ride into the canyon.

Adam needed to return to his life in Tucson and it was time for Debbie's arrival. I waited for her plane anxiously anticipating my reunion with Debbie. I had been without her only a week and even though I had thoroughly appreciated the things I had done and seen, I missed Debbie and looked forward to sharing the next week with her.

Debbie looked fantastic as she stepped into the airport terminal and I was overwhelmed with the instant desire I felt to take her in my arms. She allowed me a quick hug but then pushed me back and told me she had to tell me something.

She had wrecked her truck on the drive down to the airport. She appeared unhurt but she did have a bruise on her chest where the seat belt had squeezed her upon impact. She said that the accident occurred on the exit ramp of the interstate highway as she neared the Charlotte airport. She insisted the accident was not her fault as the driver in front of her had slammed on the brakes for no reason she could see. Now I am not now nor would I care to be an insurance adjuster but there was something a little fishy going on here. Debbie probably had approached the exit moving too quickly or she may have just been unaware of traffic in front of her. In either case, she was well. Fortunately, she had been able to call her brother who lives nearby and she did not miss her flight. I asked her to drive more slowly and take more care in the future and we left the Salt Lake terminal, had dinner and retired to a hotel room I had rented for the night. The wreck was forgotten in the joy of our reunion. I might have made a connection between Debbie's wreck and the continuing growth of necrotic tissue in Debbie's brain, but I didn't.

We spent the next eight days camping and hiking throughout the Canyonlands and Arches National Parks. We walked along canyon rims for miles, our minds staggered by the immensity of our country and the beauty of the rocks. One evening we were privy to a gathering of mule deer at the edge of the canyon rim. We walked and climbed and there was no sign at all that Debbie was struggling.

One cloudy afternoon we hiked to the Delicate Arch. This arch is famous and is pictured on every Utah license plate. Debbie was entranced and we settled in for a quiet afternoon. Soon it began to rain. This was not unpleasant as July temperatures hover near one hundred degrees. As the rain passed we saw a sight neither of us will ever forget. A rainbow appeared directly over the arch and its rays passed directly through the arch. We howled in pure delight and then a second rainbow appeared paralleling the first. We were witness to a double rainbow over the Delicate Arch!

Each day we explored different sections of the park. We began the Devil's Garden trail at sunrise, a ten mile round trip that allows marvelous vistas of many arches and the ability to climb upon them, and did not return to our campsite until darkness had fallen. We cavorted up and down the Double "O", and had lunch in the shadow of a massive red rock spire. We would sit for a while and then adjust our position every fifteen minutes or so to maintain the shade the spire afforded from the relentless sun.

One morning we drove to town and joined in a raft trip on the Colorado River. Our guide encouraged us to leave the raft and to float lazily in the river on our own. We finished that day with an exploration and a climb of the Double Arch, the same one seen in the introduction to one of the Indiana Jones movies. Some nights after our dinner we would wander the landscape near our campsite and would sit neath a rock wall or in the middle of an arch and watch the brilliance of the stars as they rotated through the sky. It was a marvelous trip and we both were sad that I had to return Debbie to Salt Lake for her return flight and that I had to begin my drive eastward.

We returned home and to our respective jobs. I went to see the damage on Debbie's truck and to retrieve her personal belongings from it. The truck was totaled. The front end was crumpled and I thanked God that Debbie or anyone else had not been injured. We purchased an old Honda that one of Debbie's co-workers had used as a second vehicle and Debbie was back on the road and back on the job.

The doctors were now more concerned about the necrosis than they had shown at first. The frequency of Debbie's MRI's was increased to once monthly. When necrotic tissue first began to appear on the MRI's we were glad that it was just necrosis and not tumorous. As the necrotic tissue continued to expand we were informed that if it did not stop its continuous buildup it could become life threatening. The necrosis is formed by the clotting of blood within the brain. The bleeding had been caused by the mega doses of radiation energy that Debbie had endured during her stereotactic radiosurgery of two summers before. It was hoped that the bleeding would stop on its own, but it did not. Debbie was suffering hundreds of tiny strokes and if they continued there would be serious deleterious effects. Dr. Desjardins began some serious research into methods of stopping this internal bleeding.

By late summer it was clear on the scans that the bleeding, despite the steroid program, was continuing. Debbie was still feeling and acting strong. She did not miss any work and still joined me on most weekends for our usual walks along the Blue Ridge. The folks at Duke decided that another biopsy was called for and Debbie agreed to undergo the procedure once more. Neither one of us was pleased with the thought of Debbie being placed inside a halo once again, but we agreed that the doctors needed to know with exact precision what was inside before they could address a way of treatment.

We returned the night prior to the scheduled operation and this time when the neurosurgeon arrived at six in the morning he examined Debbie and even though the halo and its accompanying toolbox of screwdriver and screws was at hand the doctor decided that because he had already been in Debbie's head once before he would not need the halo to guide him in this morning's procedure. This biopsy procedure went more smoothly because of this.

The pathology report came back with good news and bad news. The good news was Debbie continued to be tumor free- the bad news was the necrosis was continuing to eat up Debbie's brain. This was so hard for us to comprehend as Debbie maintained an active schedule and did not appear to be affected.

Dr. Desjardins had determined that there was a course of potential treatment. This was called Hyperbaric Chamber Treatment and would entail Debbie being inserted into a chamber where the oxygen levels would be enhanced and she would be subjected to a higher atmospheric pressure. The theory is that the extra pressure and oxygen would force the oxygen into the brain where it would encourage the sealing of the broken capillaries that were spilling their blood droplets into the cavity of Debbie's brain. The doctor's only question was when Debbie would begin these treatments.

As the year's end approached Debbie and I had made plans to visit my family in the New York area for Thanksgiving and to visit with her family for Christmas. We also planned to combine our New York trip with some concerts and were looking forward to welcoming the New Year by attending a concert in Asheville by what had become one of our favorite bands- moe. The doctor assured us that waiting until January should not be problematic and it was agreed that Debbie would begin her hyperbaric program at the beginning of 2006. In retrospect I do regret the decision to postpone the treatments. The extra month we waited may have changed the future we are now dealing with. It was Debbie's continued vibrancy that had us fooled.

Our Thanksgiving trip was fabulous. We spent three days in the Pennsylvania Dutch region and enjoyed our wanderings through the craft and antique stores of those strangely yet delightfully named towns of Blue Ball, Paradise and Intercourse. We went on to New York and after visiting with my family and eating like pigs for a couple days we attended two nights of concerts held at the historic Roseland Dance Hall. Debbie danced along with all the rest of the crowd and we walked the streets of the city afterwards enjoying the bright lights and stopping in for slices of pizza at Famous Ray's. We made love that weekend; we haven't ever since.

By the middle of December it had become obvious that Debbie was having difficulties due to the advancing necrosis. She was still rising early to go to work but was having difficulty driving her car in a straight line as she backed down our driveway. I began driving her to work on my way to school. I explained to her this was to help save money as gas prices rose to astronomical levels but it was really because I had finally become concerned about her safety behind the wheel. December is a slow month for Debbie's landscaping and she spent most of the month in her office preparing designs for the upcoming season. She worked full-time until the end of the year. We fully expected Debbie to receive her hyperbaric treatments and return to work in late March.

We spent a few days at Christmas with Debbie's family in Florida. I was now a fully accepted member of the Clark clan and we enjoyed the sunshine. We drove back to North Carolina and stayed at our friend Tamra's home in Asheville as we settled in for a three-day run of concerts. Debbie had noticeably weakened since the previous month and her gallivanting nonchalantly through the streets of New York City. She now needed assistance when taking a flight of stairs or when stepping off a curb.

At the first night's concert Debbie fell midway during the second set. This was her first fall ever and she was embarrassed to have had it happen in public. We went the next two nights to the shows but we did not try to get near the stage and we did not dance. We found seats near the back of the arena and enjoyed the shows but we both knew the beginning of this New Year did not bring the hope that a new beginning should.

CHAPTER 24

Debbie's case was now in the cutting edge of medical technology. Although still a brain cancer patient the issue we were now being forced to address, the necrosis, had been caused by the stereotactic radiosurgery she had undergone two years previously. It had taken that long for the damage to manifest itself in a way that caused physical symptoms to appear. It was still within the realms of possibility that Debbie's tumor would reoccur. It had not, but the efforts to ensure the tumor's continued absence had now caused another situation that was equally life threatening.

Did this mean, as Dr. Friedman had intimated, that the stereotactic radiosurgery was not effective. Well, yes it did. But on the other hand, no it didn't. The purpose of the radiosurgery was to destroy and eliminate the tumor and it is quite possible that it did exactly that. The tumor itself has not returned ever since the radiosurgery of 2003. It may return and appear with Debbie's next MRI but it has not come back yet.

Our doctors in 2003 told us in good faith what their opinion was as to best treatment options. We understood that there was not much history of other patients having undergone the radiosurgery procedure, as the technology did not exist long prior to its being used on Debbie. We chose it at the time because of its relatively non-invasive nature and the great potential it had shown among the small group of patients it had been tested on. We understood then that Debbie was entitled to squeal like a guinea pig, for indeed she was still engaging herself in what was a new and little used method of treatment. Unfortunately for Debbie, the procedure has caused much damage in the long run.

We could have bitched about the damage done but we understood that none of us, doctors included, are prescient. It is impossible to predict what the results of any treatment will be. For two years following the radiosurgery Debbie was as healthy and active as any cancer patient has a right to be. We hoped to have this continue forever, it didn't, but we are not bitter about that. Our goal, as always, has been to face whatever dilemma has been presented us and to maintain as happy an existence as we can. There is no use in crying over spilled milk and neither is there any advantage in regretting a past decision to the detriment of making decisions in the present.

Debbie's case record is now part of the history of medical research and because of the side effects (the necrosis) the radiosurgery had caused her, other patients will now have a better chance of determining the best treatment when they are faced with the issues of reoccurring brain tumors as Debbie has been.

Debbie was now stepping further into the realms of medical history. Since so few had ever undergone radiosurgery to halt a recurring tumor Debbie had now become one of the first to suffer necrosis as a side effect and was about to become one of the first to attempt hyperbarics as a method to curb that necrosis.

To further illustrate the concept of the cutting edge of Debbie's treatment I relate this story that also demonstrates the attributes of a great physician working in a patient-first environment. One evening I answered the phone and it was Dr. Desjardins. The doctor was calling from an out of town conference and after checking that we were fine she mentioned that she had just heard of a new medicine that would enhance the effect of the steroids in stopping the internal bleeding. She said that the results in the test group were promising- a 60% or three of five success rate. I agreed this sounded quite promising. "Three of five", I remember repeating. The doctor said I should not get too excited as three of five meant exactly that. Debbie became the sixth person to ever try that particular drug for the purpose of halting internal bleeding in the brain.

Our problem now was logistical. There are no facilities locally for Debbie to undergo the hyperbaric treatments she needed. We had been informed of a facility in Charlotte and arranged with Debbie's brother for her to stay with him and for Debbie to drive the seven miles from his home just across the NC-SC state line to downtown Charlotte where the facility was located. I would bring Debbie down there and make sure the treatments were begun before returning to my job. I would return to Charlotte and stay with Debbie every weekend during the twelve weeks the treatments would take. Debbie was scheduled to receive sixty treatments, one every weekday. Each treatment would take between 3-4 hours.

It was explained to Debbie that the forced introduction of oxygen to her brain was integral to the closing of the still bleeding capillaries. It was further explained that cigarette smoking reduces oxygen levels and would be completely counter-productive to what we were trying to achieve. Debbie, who had been a two and a half pack a day smoker for over twenty-five years, quit cold turkey on New Years Eve. She smoked her final cigarette before retiring to bed.

CHAPTER 25

Debbie and I met with Dr. "H" in her office a few days following New Year's. Dr. "H" explained that Debbie would need to disrobe completely and not wear anything but a hospital gown when she was placed in the chamber. Debbie could not bring anything into the chamber with her. No books, no magazines, no nothing. Debbie would even have to remove her wedding ring. The reason for this was that because of the high intensity of oxygen in the chamber any spark could cause a flash fire similar to the one that killed three Apollo astronauts on the launch pad. We signed the usual papers allowing treatment to be performed and accepting the potential side effects which included bursting eardrums, rupture of the sinuses, blindness and of course that old standby- death. Dr. "H" also told us that Debbie would need to present herself at least thirty minutes prior to her scheduled treatment time and that if she was ever late treatment for that day would be cancelled although it would still be billed. Debbie eventually received sixty treatments at the Charlotte facility. She actually saw Dr. "H" only one more time.

The following morning I drove Debbie for her first treatment. We met the hyperbaric nurse who told us we would not be able to receive treatment that day, as the insurance had not as yet approved the procedure. This made me livid. The arrangements for the treatment and all insurance papers had been forwarded over a month before. There was no further reason for any delay. Debbie was debilitating daily. Her strength was rapidly deteriorating.

A social worker was brought in to speak with us and see if we could cut the bureaucratic red tape. The hyperbaric nurse told us there was nothing Dr. "H" could do. I knew better as I had already seen that the insurance companies just needed to be told by a doctor that the treatment being prescribed is the best treatment to cure the ills of the patient. The social worker, although kind and polite, was essentially useless. She did not have the medical authority to confront the insurance people and the only reason she was really called was to get us out of the hospital without a scene.

I borrowed the telephone and called Dr. Desjardins. Within the hour the payment issue was settled and Debbie's first appointment was rescheduled for the next day. We were not offered any compensation for the morning we spent wasting our time and dissipating Debbie's remaining energies. I was also amazed several months later when the bills began to find their way to our house. Dr. "H" who had trouble fighting on behalf of Debbie had no problem at all in charging an exorbitant amount for personal services. The doctor claimed a fee of $3000 for each and every one of the sixty treatments despite not appearing once in the treatment room. This bill was in addition to the one charged by the hospital for the use of the facility and the performance of the hyperbaric technician. The doctor did perform a physical examination of Debbie at the completion of the thirtieth treatment in her office. As you can see Dr. "H" was one of the few doctors we have met not worthy of the title and not worthy of our respect.

The first treatment happened with a bit of apprehension. We were afraid that Debbie would not react well to the increased pressure of the chamber and were concerned that something could go wrong if her body was unable to tolerate it.

The chamber itself resembles a torpedo tube just large enough to allow the width of a single bed inside. The bed itself was on rollers that slid out from the tube that was made of clear, thick reinforced plastic. It was explained that there was no glass as it might easily shatter under the extreme pressure. Debbie lie upon the bed and the bed was slid inside the tube. The whole thing sealed with a door that resembled the hatch on a submarine. You sealed it shut by tightening a wheel. It was told to us that if there were an emergency it would take several minutes for the pressure to be released to the point where the door could be unlocked. We were told that if the door were to be opened without the pressure being released then the chamber, with Debbie in it, would burst through the drywall of the room we were in and not settle until it was several hundred feet down the corridor.

Debbie was helped onto the bed by the technician. She was a woman our age and did do a wonderful job in making Debbie as comfortable as she could be. The bed was placed inside and we checked the intercom system. All was well, we could hear Debbie and she could hear us. Debbie was reminded to continue swallowing as the pressure rose within the chamber and to holler and signal if she was feeling any undue discomfort. The technician said she would begin raising the pressure in very small increments so that if Debbie was experiencing a problem we would be able to get her out quicker. The pressure switch was flipped and a hiss of air could be heard. Debbie gave us a thumbs up and the pressure continued to rise until the prescribed level was reached. Debbie was fine and asked if she could now watch the television that was suspended above the chamber. She could and she calmly watched Animal Planet for the next several hours. I stayed the entire time occasionally speaking with Debbie on the intercom, occasionally making faces at her inside the tube. She did not sleep during that first treatment but Debbie did become so tolerant of the procedure that she did catch some catnaps at later treatments. At the end of the allotted time the nurse began to slowly release the pressure from the chamber. This took nearly half an hour as it was imperative to return Debbie to normal pressure slowly otherwise Debbie would suffer the "bends".

I was glad I had decided to stay to make sure treatments had begun before I returned back up the mountain and to my students. It had been an extremely frustrating few days but I felt good knowing that Debbie would be safe and that I would see her again on Friday evening.

After the first week Debbie began complaining of some hearing problems. The nurse consulted with Dr. "H" and it was determined that Debbie would be required to have a tiny hole punched through her eardrum and to have a drain placed there. This would alleviate the pressure from inside the ear and allow Debbie to continue the hyperbaric program. An appointment with an ear specialist was made and the procedure was performed. Debbie returned to her treatments and did not suffer any other ill effects.

Debbie did at this time begin to complain of great fatigue. She blamed it on the treatments but the real reason was the continued bleeding in her head. No one who has met Debbie for the first time after the fall of 2005 ever has had the opportunity to meet the active and vivacious workhorse of a woman that Debbie had been.

Another problem developed in Debbie's second week of treatments. I received a call at school from the hyperbaric nurse. Debbie had not made it to her appointment that morning. I called her brother's home and no one there was at home either. Brad and Tina, Debbie's brother and niece, were at work. I took a break every half hour to return to the school office and use the phone. I was frantic. Finally as my day neared dismissal, Debbie answered the phone. She was fine; she had just gotten lost on her way to the hospital. Remember, Debbie had been making the trip now nearly ten times and the way should have been imprinted. The necrosis was now affecting her mentally as well as physically and it was even more important she complete the hyperbaric program.

I also now and belatedly understood that Debbie could no longer be trusted at all behind the wheel of a car. I also understood I would have to return to Charlotte immediately and arrange transportation plans for Debbie to be taken to the hospital daily. My principal had been standing nearby monitoring my side of the phone conversation and he understood my need. I was told to take off as long as I needed. I could not be paid for my missed days but my job was secure. I left the building, returned home to gather up D.D. the Dog and drove back down the mountain to Charlotte.

I drove Debbie to the hospital the next morning and assisted the nurse in preparing Debbie for the chamber. While Debbie was inside I met once again with the social worker. We went through every possible method of transport available and kept coming to the same roadblock. Debbie was staying at her brother's home in Tega Cay, a small town just south of the state line. His house was less than one mile from the actual state borderline. The ambulances and medical transport vehicles could not cross state lines because somewhere, someone at sometime had said they couldn't. We could not get any one to budge. The only option was a private car service that was willing to transport Debbie for a round trip of forty dollars a day. This would have to be paid daily and in cash. The insurance would not cover this because it was not considered a medical transport. An ambulance would be medical transport but the ambulances would not cross the line. This was a classic Catch 22.

I knew we were in trouble because there was no way I would be able to afford to pay for a car service. I didn't even need a calculator to do the math. $40 a day became $200 a week, became $800 a month. My take home pay, as an experienced schoolteacher at state scale was approximately $2200 a month. The real problem was that with Debbie not working anymore her health insurance had been transferred to Cobra. The payments to maintain Debbie's insurance were close to $1800 a month. I was really taking home a bit over $300 and it was just barely covering the gas back and forth from Charlotte. I was dipping into our meager savings just to stay afloat.

We had applied in December for Social Security disability on Debbie's behalf. The folks at the Brain Tumor Center had helped to gather the necessary documents to support Debbie's case but we were told that even if Debbie would be approved (she was) there was a two-year waiting period before benefits would be paid out and before Medicare would take over her insurance. This meant Cobra for the next two years, otherwise Debbie would be denied any treatments including the basic MRI scans that had monitored her condition and had alerted us several times already to problems. There was no money to pay for transport. No one was available to drive Debbie on a daily basis and Debbie could no longer safely get to the hospital. Well, if Debbie can't get to the hospital, then the hospital will have to get closer to Debbie.

Debbie's nephew Jeremy lived within the city limits of Charlotte on the correct side of the state line. He was living with his fiancée Christine and I approached them with our dilemma. If Debbie could stay with you we could access a volunteer Red Cross driver to take Debbie daily to and from the hospital. Christine immediately said something for which I will always love her and be in her debt, "Family comes first".

For the next two and a half months Debbie stayed with Jeremy and Christine and they allowed me to visit every weekend. We had wonderful times together listening to music and watching sports together on TV. We made a tradition of having Sunday brunch out and generally did our best of making a terrible situation better.

Jeremy has since become a marathon runner and Christine is now the mother of two. We love them and can never repay their kindness.

Debbie completed the round of sixty treatments and came back home to me in late April. The MRI taken upon the conclusion of the program showed a clear cavity and the white ghostly lines that represented the necrotic tissue were gone. It seemed that the hyperbaric chamber had done its job. Now we could only wait and see if Debbie's strength would return.

Sadly we were forced to inform Debbie's employers that she would be physically unable to return to work. The truth was Debbie could hardly walk and a physical therapy program was started immediately so that she could relearn that very basic skill we all take for granted.

CHAPTER 26

The relationship between Debbie and I while remaining a loving one has become more one-sided. Debbie now had needs well beyond the ordinary. She really did need help every time she attempted to step outside the front door of our house. Her walking gait had become a disaster. She would place her right foot, her whole body would lean to the right, and then her left foot would slide forward an inch or two while scraping the ground. In this manner Debbie could meticulously cover about a hundred feet in approximately fifteen minutes. That is if her stamina would allow her to remain upright for fifteen minutes without crumpling to the ground.

We were told that the neural pathways that controlled her left side had been destroyed by the advance of the necrotic tissue. Although still a brain cancer patient Debbie now resembled a stroke victim with semi-paralysis of one side of her body. We were also told that neurons (nerves, if you prefer) could not be reattached once they were severed. This would seem to mean that Debbie would never have the ability to walk normally again. This is not so. It is possible through usage and practice for the brain to develop new pathways. In effect, if Debbie could be taught to walk again somehow and practiced that new skill constantly, the brain would rewire itself and Debbie would be able to walk. This was the goal of the intensive physical therapy program.

This was really so sad. To compare Debbie of 2006 with the Debbie of the previous year was enough to bring tears to my eyes. It was so disheartening to watch her as she struggled to walk down a corridor her left foot never leaving the floor. Walks of a hundred yards literally were as tiresome to Debbie as hikes of fifteen miles had once been. Debbie would have to lie down and rest after every exertion.

I was instructed to encourage Debbie to raise her foot with every step. The only chance Debbie would have to walk normally depended upon her ability to overcome the necrosis, and to be able to move her leg upon command. She could not do it. Spring became summer and Debbie was still unable to control her own leg.

We still went outdoors as often as my schedule and the weather would allow. We would go to overlooks on the Blue Ridge Parkway and Debbie would hobble over a few yards from the car and we would sit contentedly in the grass having our picnic lunches. Debbie would allow me to wander off a bit on my own and I would stretch my own legs by hustling into the woods for a quick 20-30 minute round trip. I never have, and still don't, feel comfortable leaving Debbie alone like that but it remains the only way for me to retain any sort of muscle tone. I would snap pictures of everything I saw so that I could share the images with Debbie later. I made sure to take pictures of any interesting flowers I came across.

The command to "lift your foot" quickly became monotonous. You would think that having heard it thousands of times Debbie would internalize that command and begin to lift her foot. If you thought such a thing, why, you would be mistaken. We began though to see a small difference after each reminder. Debbie would be trying to lift her foot and although that difference was miniscule at first there was a difference when Debbie was reminded.

One day after several months and thousands of attempts Katherine, Debbie's physical therapist, screamed delightedly that Debbie had lifted her left foot off of the ground. This was a symbolic and monumental step forward and with work and practice would actually become a forward moving step. It did show that some neural pathways were finding other ways to reattach themselves within Debbie's brain. In another two weeks or so Debbie had achieved a full step in which her left foot did lift off the ground and set itself in front of her right foot. It now became Debbie's mission to repeat that tens of thousands of times reinforcing the strength of her newly developed neural pathway.

Although Debbie has never been able to walk smoothly as she did prior to the development of the necrosis she finally was able to put the parts of a reasonable walking stride together. She developed the ability to walk again for longer distances and soon we were able to extend our outdoor activities to include walks of up to a half-mile. Debbie would tire frequently but I was more than willing to accommodate her and would help her to sit comfortably on the forest floor and then help her to stand when she was ready to start anew.

None of this came about easily. It was all so slow and painstaking. Debbie had been like a mountain goat able to cavort and play comfortably in any wilderness situation. Now it was all she could do to walk on a level path for a short distance. It would have to be enough; it was all there was.

It was during this time that I found myself forced to place some restrictions on Debbie. I was going to work and leaving her to fend for herself until the late afternoon when I could return home. There were several occasions I would find Debbie lying in the yard or on the floor indoors unable to get up. She could never tell me with precision how long she had been prostrate. She always claimed it had just happened. I began to insist she remain indoors while I was away. I also had to forbid her from using our oven or stovetop while I was at work. She had developed the very disturbing habit of forgetting that she was cooking and I would discover scorched pans. We were quite lucky she did not start a fire.

Debbie was making progress. She was getting stronger a little bit at a time and we could measure her progress every time we went out on a trail. We would rejoice every time Debbie would go further than she had before. Walks of 100 feet, lengthened to a hundred yards, then to a few hundred yards, then to a half-mile and by the end of the summer Debbie had successfully accomplished trail walks of a complete mile. These walks would take us entire afternoons, but neither of us had anything better to do. Seeing the progress she was making allowed Debbie to feel triumphant and she continued to build on her success and this in turn allowed her to develop new neural pathways that would ensure further success.

This march toward progress came to an abrupt halt with the reading of Debbie's October MRI. Bleeding had begun again inside Debbie's head. It was determined that the only thing was to have Debbie undergo another series of sixty hyperbaric treatments.

We refused to return to Charlotte, as we had never been satisfied with Dr. "H". It would also have been too much to ask of Jeremy and Christine. They were in the process of renovating their house with intent to sell. Debbie would have been uncomfortable amid all the construction and she would have been in the way. We researched the locations of other hyperbaric chambers and discovered that one was located in Sarasota, Florida. Debbie's sister Jennifer lives in Sarasota and Debbie's mother resides just a half-hour south of there. We elected to have Debbie stay with her mom. Debbie's mom and her older brother Dean would be able to transport Debbie daily and Jennifer could help out when necessary.

It was arranged that Debbie would begin her treatments the week of Thanksgiving. This was ideal as it coincided with the days off I would receive from school. We packed Debbie's stuff and I drove her to Florida. The first day of orientation in Sarasota went smoothly. We met with the male nurse/technician who would be administering the treatments. He was wonderfully friendly and considerate and we shared similar interests in music. I felt greatly reassured and comfortable that Debbie would be treated with care and gentleness. The chamber itself was similar and Debbie was experienced in accepting the claustrophobic nature of the hyperbaric tube. The second series of sixty treatments were underway.

I returned home to a cold house. It was lonely, yes, but it was also quite literally cold. Our oil furnace had broken down and needed a replacement. I reached into our savings once more to deal with this emergency. Unfortunately it took several weeks for the new furnace to be shipped and delivered and I spent a frigid month alone. I was calling Debbie nightly and getting updates from her mother as well. I was looking forward to Christmas so that I could spend the time with Debbie and to be warm.

Debbie and I had a wonderful Christmas week together. I had found a good price on a hotel room for the week and Debbie and I stayed alone allowing her mother a respite from Debbie care. I would take Debbie to the hospital and then we would walk slowly along one of the many beaches on the Gulf Coast. We discovered an inexpensive family seafood restaurant and tried many different varieties of fish we had never had before.

There were some issues to attend to. Debbie's mom had broken her wrist and was uncomfortable driving Debbie. Her brother Dean had suffered a traumatic stabbing incident at the hands of his ex-wife and his life was shattered. He had moved in with his mom but he was unable to lay off the bottle of vodka that became an ever-present accompaniment to his fashion sense. Debbie told me she was afraid to allow him to drive her anymore, as he was always drunk. Dean had always been an outgoing and caring individual but the demons that had led him to the bottle were too strong for him to overcome.

Once again, Debbie was moved in the middle of her treatments. This time it was to her sister Jen's. Once again, the Red Cross was enlisted to transport Debbie to and from the hospital. The volunteers who accompanied Debbie daily were magnificent and totally reliable.

New Year's Eve passed quietly. I was forced to return home and work. I was lonely every single day. It was expected that Debbie's treatment would continue until mid-February and I made arrangements to drive back to Florida and pick up Debbie over a three-day weekend our school schedule had conveniently provided.

Debbie was once again weak, as she did not engage in the stamina building activities that I insisted upon. We were glad she was home though and now that the new furnace was installed and working properly Debbie never had to suffer any cold days that entire winter.

CHAPTER 27

I sat and talked with an elderly gentleman yesterday afternoon while waiting for Debbie to complete her physical therapy session. He had a walker to assist him but his mind and sense of humor were apparently quite clear. He called to me from across the lobby and as I sat down alongside him he asked if it would be all right to ask me a question. Of course, I responded and he then asked me how long I have worn my beard. I proceeded to tell him how I had undergone back surgery in the mid-nineties to repair a ruptured disc in my spine and how for the weeks of recovery I lay flat on my back and by the time I had recovered enough to stand and walk comfortably my beard had become a fait accompli. He then asked me if it helped me get any ass. I cracked up at the incongruity of the question but answered him honestly by saying that it hadn't hurt my chances at first but that it didn't seem to be doing me any good recently. I explained that my courtship with Debbie took place a year after I had grown it but that since her relapse at the end of 2005 I hadn't got any. He told me I had suffered through more than my share of bad luck but that he respected me as a man.

We went on and he spoke about the shamefulness of politicians willing to line the pockets of corporate interests at the expense of people like us. He lamented his requiring a walker when he had once been such a physically active individual. He explained how he had once been a professional athlete having risen to the "AAA" level of baseball's minor leagues. We spoke about what happens to us after we die. We agreed that neither of the two of us knew the answer to that one but that for some reason beyond our comprehension, we are hopeful. It was a short conversation that didn't last fifteen minutes but its impact upon me has been a powerful one.

That man is me ten or fifteen years from now. My body will continue aging and I will need the support of the Social Security benefits that I have contributed toward my entire life. Otherwise I will not have the benefit of a walker when I need it nor will I have the opportunity to engage in professional physical therapy sessions. I will fall once and be lucky if someone assists me before I starve to death lying on the floor. Do I sound crazy? I think not. My newfound friend and Debbie too have been fortunate to live in a country where compassion for our sick and elderly has been built into our social fabric. That fabric is rapidly unraveling before our eyes and I wonder what will happen to people as they age in the future. The sick and aged have not and will never be able to contribute to the economic machine- will they be cared for? Will you be cared for? Your parents? That funny old man I met yesterday is all of us.

My future is bleak. Debbie is ill and although she continues to maintain, I still live in daily fear that any morning may be her last. My own body has begun to show age. My eyesight is erratic at best during the glare of the afternoon. My blood pressure is high and my teeth are horrendous. I have no health insurance at all for myself. No private company is willing to touch me without demanding a premium that is far in excess of what I can afford. I cannot go to work, as then there would be no one to care for Debbie. I stand by my choice to care for Debbie, it is the right and moral thing to do and secondarily my effort is saving society the cost of Debbie's care. But, it is sacrificing my future.

How will you decide when faced with these issues of aging and health? You'd better think twice because you will be. Of course, maybe aging won't affect you- maybe you are the only living member in the entire history of the human race that will not grow old and eventually die. Maybe, just don't count on it.

CHAPTER 28

It was fabulous to have Debbie home again for the spring of 2007. The previous year had seen Debbie living away from home for half the year. She had spent the winter and spring in Charlotte and then the late fall and early winter in Florida in order to accommodate the hyperbaric treatments that so far have halted the life threatening internal bleeding of her brain.

She continued for the next year on a one month MRI schedule. Each month we held our breath for a day or two while we awaited the report on her most current scan. Each month we breathed a bit easier as the scans continued to show that the hyperbarics had, for the moment, shut down the leakage of blood into Debbie's brain cavity.

It would have been great had the halting of the bleeding corresponded with Debbie's regaining her ability to walk and maintain her balance. This was not so. Debbie did through extreme effort on her part regain some of her previous ability to walk, but it was now clear to any who passed us on a flat trail or in a park, that Debbie was struggling. In addition, some of the mental capacities we take for granted were slipping away from Debbie. I could no longer count on her being able to restrain her impulse control.

Debbie would seem to be doing well, when suddenly she would lurch forward to reach for something and she would fall. We were taught by the doctor and by her physical therapist to discuss the cause and possible prevention of each and every fall. Invariably Debbie would say that there was something she wanted and she went to get it. I would ask what and she would say it was a leaf on one of our houseplants that needed to be pruned, or a napkin she dropped, or a bead she needed for her next project, or a speck of dirt that needed cleaning. Debbie's response could be anything, it didn't really matter, and it was always something small and relatively unimportant. I tried to stress to Debbie that she needed to ask for help as none of these things were worth her taking an unnecessary fall. She would agree and nod her head, but the next time she had a whim to do something, she would not ask for assistance and she would be on the ground again. Debbie was totally unable to think through an action and analyze its potential risk. If she thought she needed something, her impulsive behavior took charge every time. She suffered many falls.

I was working still. The students in my care were children who had been through difficult times of their own. Almost all of them had been sexually assaulted by a trusted grownup. All of them had inflicted a sexual assault upon another child. They had been through the court system and been found by a judge to be dangerous to society and in need of psychological care to help them overcome their trauma. These children were profane and violent. It was common in our school to hear the outbursts of four letter words sometimes coupled with actual attacks upon fellow students, teachers or supporting staff. The procedure I pursued was to allow a cooling off period to be followed by a calm and logical discussion of what had caused the outburst. I was amazed at the logic the children were able to indulge in. Although their acts were near insane the reasons for their acts actually made sense. I found that if I could acknowledge their reasoning and present alternate methods for them to achieve their goals I could significantly lower the frequency of violence in my classroom. It was in the use of logic that I could reach my students and help them move forward in their goals of returning to their homes and communities and being released from the control of the justice system. I was thoroughly distraught that at home Debbie would not respond to logic at all.

Debbie would be on the ground rubbing the sore butt caused by her latest fall, yet she would continue to insist that the picture needed straightening. No amount of cajoling or begging on my part has ever been able to convince Debbie that her fall was preventable had she only asked for help or if she had waited until she could ask for help when I returned from work. Her logic could not accommodate anything other than seeing or wanting something and then proceeding thoughtlessly to achieve what she wanted.

Sometimes I would see Debbie about to do something potentially hazardous. I would ask her to stop, she wouldn't. Sometimes she would fall, but sometimes she wouldn't. This was even worse than the falling because it falsely gave her the confidence to continue with her next impulsive act that would then cause a fall. This repetition began to fray my nerves. I care and did not wish Debbie to hurt herself but my warnings were unheeded and the logic of thinking through an action before rushing to do it was ignored. I was having more success at school than I was at home.

Debbie did begin a new phase to her artistic creativity. She had been stymied by her physical inability to continue to work safely in our yard and flowerbeds. Debbie needed some outlet to occupy her time and so she developed an interest in beading and jewelry making. I purchased supplies for her at a local craft store and Debbie began spending hours a day in her easy chair meticulously counting and stringing beads. Her first efforts were childlike but she did accept some artistic criticism from me. I had once worked in a necklace shop where I learned how to create jewelry so my advice had some foundation. Debbie tried some things I had suggested and liked the results. She began a whirlwind of beading and had soon produced over a hundred different necklaces and bracelets. The pieces I liked the best were free-form mobiles she created using beads with sticks that she would gather when on our short walks in the woods. Over the next few years Debbie has graciously gifted many of our friends and relatives with pieces she has created. None of these items has any real commercial value but they do symbolize Debbie's love for the person so gifted.

The seasons passed quickly enough. We continued to maintain our schedule of walks through the woods and forests of the Blue Ridge. Debbie's walking, although clearly unbalanced, was quantum leaps better than it had been. She could lift her left foot and was able to place it in front of her right. She could maintain a continuous stride, right foot, left foot and repeat interminably. Sometimes Debbie would freeze up and her left side would begin to quiver. Usually a verbal cue to lift her foot would get her moving again. Other times I would have to provide additional support and either hold her hand or to place a strong hand in the small of her back to get her moving again.

Debbie would freeze up at things we used to just walk right past without a second's notice. A small twig in the path could cause Debbie to stop dead in her tracks. It was frightening to see her freeze and be totally unable to move. You could see her effort in trying to will her body to respond to her mind's commands and the emotional stress it was causing her to be completely stuck. All we could do was to get her started again in any way possible and continue until the next time.

Our walks began to wear me down completely. It is physically challenging to me to walk at Debbie's slow pace. It also caused me physical pain to use my strength to support her weight, to push her to start again when she froze and to lift her when she fell.

Many times friends would visit and would join us on one of Debbie's walks. No matter how hard they tried to keep up with Debbie, they were always thirty feet ahead without even being aware they had left us in the dust. I would call to them and they would turn disbelieving how far behind them we had fallen. They were sincerely trying to walk with Debbie; they just couldn't walk that slowly.

Debbie's walks have become an ongoing test of her strength and stamina. We can always measure her progress, or lack thereof, by how far we can get on any given trail or path. I made sure that we never attempted anything that would find us stranded too far from our vehicle and always encouraged Debbie to rest and conserve her strength for the return trip. Many times we turned around and headed back early if Debbie felt at all uncomfortable about her ability to get back safely

I also made sure that Debbie took the time during our outdoor excursions to just relax and enjoy the beauty and solitude of the mountains and forests. I allowed her to linger at any site she felt was particularly beautiful or that had a peculiar flower that she could examine closer. She needed to be reminded to look around frequently as her effort in maintaining her balance as she walked required all her attention. Many times I would point things out to her for her perusal- things she would have easily noticed in the past without missing a stride. The amazing thing was that when we stopped and Debbie had rested she would then become the person pointing items of interest out to me.

Debbie's determination to remain active allowed her to relearn how to walk. It did not prevent her falls or help with impulse control but she did learn to walk again. She had practiced enough that new neural pathways had developed. She looked out of whack when she walked, but at least she was walking.

She was also still falling. One afternoon I returned from work and found Debbie in our yard lying head facing downhill on the steep slope that borders our front yard. She was only a few feet from what would have been a severe fall of at least ten feet. She was entangled in the briars of this unkempt portion of our yard and she, fortunately as it turned out, had stopped struggling to pick herself up and just lay with the blood rushing to her head waiting for me to return from work and help her back up. Other than a few scratches on her arms from the briars she was unhurt. I helped her up and back inside but I was shocked. Debbie had avoided serious injury, but not by much. Her impulse control had failed her once more. She had seen a piece of trash that had blown underneath the evergreen tree that stood sentinel over our yard and went to retrieve it when she fell and began rolling down the hill toward the unprotected slope. She almost fell to what would have been certain injury for a lousy, stinking piece of trash.

I knew that I couldn't really continue to count on Debbie to maintain her own safety anymore. I didn't really know what to do. We could not afford someone to baby-sit her every day that I went to work. I could not allow her to be placed in a rest home where she would be safe but where her independence would be removed and where her mobility would be limited to walking an interior corridor for the remainder of her life. I just couldn't do that to her.

Debbie's two-year waiting period for her Social Security disability benefits had passed. She concurrently became eligible for Medicare and I would no longer be responsible for her Cobra insurance payments that had been wiping out the benefits of my paycheck anyway. Our household income would fall by a few hundred dollars a month with the change from my working to living on Debbie's disability but I could not justify the risk or the cost that Debbie being home alone could entail.

I made the decision to leave my position at work and to devote myself full-time to Debbie's care.

CHAPTER 29

I have always been a saver. Even when I was a child working for my father at his gas station I would hold onto the money I earned. I admit that on some of the hotter summer days and when I had made a pocketful of change in tips I might splurge on a chocolate milk shake when the ice cream truck came in for gas. For the most part though, I saved up my money.

This has served me in good stead throughout the years. When I was a teenager in Brooklyn having a stash of cash allowed me to join my friend Randy in purchasing season tickets to the New York Knicks at Madison Square Garden. We enjoyed five wonderful seasons together including the last championship the Knicks have enjoyed in 38 years. Perhaps the Knicks should stop wasting their money on lousy ballplayers and should return Randy and I to our seats upstairs at mid court below the announcer's booth. All sports superstitions say you should never change anything during a winning streak.

As I grew older, it was the money I saved throughout the rest of the year that allowed me to go on concert tours. It was saved money that has allowed every trip away from home I have ever taken. I had learned to live frugally in order to be able to afford those vacations and extravagances that have provided whatever adventure I have indulged in.

When Debbie and I married she carried with her a few thousand dollars in credit card debt. I had learned the hard way that credit cards are convenient, useful and potentially dangerous. I had racked up a few thousand in debt myself in the early 80's. When I came to my senses after five years of indiscriminate spending I shut down my traveling and poured all available cash into settling my accounts. The first thing I did with Debbie after our honeymoon was to aggressively wipe out her credit card debits. After this was accomplished we found that with our both working and with the double income coming in, we were doing quite well, thank you very much. I had already begun to siphon any extra cash I had into my mortgage. Now I began to double and triple our home mortgage payments.

All this bothered Debbie at first. She did not like the idea of bringing lunch and snacks from home. She had become used to spending several dollars a day in the snack and soda machines at work. When I sat down with her and she saw that she was spending over a hundred dollars a month and that we could use that money for weekend getaways instead, she changed her ways.

So, we were fortunate in our economic status when Debbie was stricken with her tumor. Our house was paid for and we no longer had a mortgage payment. This extra cash went toward quickly paying off the car loan on the new Chevy Aveo we had purchased in 2004. At the end of 2007 when Debbie became eligible for her disability payments we had no outstanding loans or debts at all. Our credit card bills were limited to our purchases at the gas pump and they were paid off in full every month. The few times when we went out to dinner, we paid cash. I hoped we would be ready for this blind jump into dependence on nothing but a benefit check, but I was afraid.

I can hear some of you grumbling that we were becoming parasites on the social welfare teat. Stop your whining now! Debbie and I both had worked our entire lives and had paid without complaint into the Social Security pool. This was in addition to our state and federal taxes. The government promised that should we ever need to make a claim on that money, God forbid we should become disabled, it would be there to tide us over. Well, Debbie is disabled and we have made a legal claim. We feel no guilt about accepting the monthly benefit. The check we receive is for $1103 per month. We live on that. It pays for everything we eat, the pills Debbie must buy, the clothes and shoes we wear, the gas that goes in our car so that we can transport Debbie to her doctor and physical therapy appointments- everything! Our house and car are paid for. I do not know how we could possibly make ends meet if we were paying rent or still had a mortgage to deal with. I do not know how others receiving their disability are able to cope.

I was very worried the first few months I wasn't working. It was clear that someone had to be with Debbie to protect her safety and we couldn't afford someone on the salary I was earning as a fully licensed and accredited teacher being paid on the state scale. The question was could we afford to have me stay at home and still be able to afford our groceries? The answer is yes, but just barely. After the first couple months of being home I was satisfied that we could get by. I was saving $50 in cash each month that I could stockpile to use for emergencies. Emergencies show up frequently. An emergency can be anything unexpected. Replacing the tires on the car easily wiped out four or five months of meticulously held back cash.

The Medicare program had also insisted that we trim our savings account back to $23,000. This was quite amusing as Debbie I did have to liquidate some cash in order to qualify. We had an overage of almost $4000 that we had to dispose of. Both our lives savings totaled a little over $27,000. When I say we have lived frugally, I am not kidding.

We did have a small cushion the first few months of my unemployment. I had actually been laid off and was entitled to unemployment benefits. The school I had worked at had become a private enterprise and they were trying to cut back on their payroll. I had seen that my time was needed at home so I arranged with my principal to be the one to be laid off. This helped save my co-workers positions for a short while.

After receiving a few months of unemployment benefits an extension for six additional months was offered to me. I refused it. Debbie's condition had worsened instead of getting better and my time at home was now needed more than ever. I had hoped that I might be able to accept a night shift or part time job and had been willing to do so. I now realized even that was out of the question and so I could not in good faith continue to accept the state offered unemployment extension. I was no longer willing to accept work, unless Debbie could be cared for whenever I was absent from home. No job offer came with the promise of home care so I opted out of the system altogether and refused the money I could have easily accepted.

Debbie's condition was failing. The hard won progress she had achieved in relearning how to walk had been wiped away with the coming of spring. Debbie was falling more than ever and the MRI scan showed us why. Debbie had suffered another internal bleed sometime during the winter months. The scan showed a bleed had occurred. It also showed that the bleeding had found a way to stop on its own. The hyperbarics had continued to do their job in limiting the damage.

Debbie was forced to relearn the steps she had mastered. Debbie was extremely distraught. I had never, until then, seen Debbie flustered by the illness she had been saddled with. Now she was emotionally unable to start back over. All the achievements of the previous years work were gone. Her left leg would not any longer respond to her willful command and she had to start again. The fact she was able to finally accept this evil fate and to again work the therapy program is a tribute to her spirit.

Debbie had other things to deal with too. She no longer had mastery of her bladder. Her mind was only able to focus on a single physical activity at a time. This meant that when she needed to pee she had to use all her willpower to rise from her chair (or bed, if it was nighttime) and walk as best as she could toward the commode. Her walk now involved the dragging of her left foot with every advance of her right. She would have to stand over the commode while unbuttoning her pants and still manage to squeeze those pelvic muscles tight while attempting to lower her panties and then sit safely upon the toilet. Many times she was unable to control that many different movements and motions at the same time and the stream of urine would escape prematurely. Similar situations sometimes, but thankfully not as frequently, would occur when she needed to have a bowel movement. At first, Debbie was too embarrassed to share these issues with me, but it was impossible to disguise the smell. We have come to accept this leakage as just another part of our daily routine. Debbie has been taught exercises that will help strengthen her pelvic squeeze and I just do an extra load of laundry. It is sad that this too has become a part of our life, but it has, and just like everything else we have been dealt, we face up to it.

We were determined, as always, to make the best of every single day. We had a few thousand dollars we had to dispose of and I no longer was involved in an active work search. We purchased a new stove and a washer and dryer. With the thousand or so still left over we decided to once again take a trip out west.

We stayed once again with my nephew Adam in Tucson. His hospitality has been fantastic. He is a very busy young man. He works at a facility that develops solar energy cells utilizing a laser technology to create the most efficient cell possible. The science of it all is beyond my understanding but we did have fun playing with a portable laser beam and creating reflections in streetlights. Adam is also an avid rock climber and a member of two different bands. He still found time to accompany Debbie and I on some of our day trips and was instrumental in helping Debbie to a precarious perch on the rocks at the Windy Point vista at Mt. Lemmon.

Most days Debbie and I would go alone and find short walks where Debbie could experience the feel of the desert without having to go too far from the car. The days of our last western vacation when Debbie walked indiscriminately through the red rocks of

Utah were gone. Every step was a struggle, but struggle on we did and we had a great time exploring new sites every day.

On our return trip east, we made stops at the Petrified Forest and at Canyon De Chelly. Debbie had seen my photos from 2005 and she wanted to see these places for herself. I was happy to accommodate her and Debbie scared the pants off me, as she would continue to inch closer to the sheer precipices of the canyons. She still had the adventurous spirit and I encouraged her to join me in leaving the safety of the fenced overlooks and wandering a hundred yards or so along the cliffs. It has always amazed me that almost all visitors to the national parks never get further from their vehicle than they can see. By just going a very short distance from the parking areas you can experience the size and immensity of our great country. Debbie could barely walk, yet she was outdoing and outperforming 98% of her countrymen.

Nowhere was this concept demonstrated more than at the Grand Canyon. We had not been there since that magical evening at the end of our honeymoon. I never thought we would ever be able to return when Debbie was stricken with her cancer. We entered the park and when confronted with the awesome spectacle of this marvelous wonder I burst into uncontrollable tears. I was overwhelmed and it took me several moments to regain my composure. Debbie and I spent a marvelous afternoon driving to the various vista points and then walking along the canyon edge until we could no longer see the overlook from which we came. If there is any place on this earth that can place your life and troubles in perspective it is while you stand at the rim of the Grand Canyon. It is a spiritual and an emotional experience. It's also just plain fun.

We drove on to Colorado Springs to see our friends Mike and Debbie. Our friendship had not diminished even though time and distance had created a barrier to our seeing each other often. We were looking forward to just relaxing with folks who knew us well and that we were completely comfortable with. Their home is located on the Front Range and the NORAD defense facility can be seen on the towering mountain behind them. The view looking east stretches for hundreds of miles across the flat plains and at night you can see the thread of the highway taking cars and people across Kansas and beyond.

Debbie and I had barely settled in for what we hoped would become a weeklong stay when we received a phone call from Debbie's mom. Debbie's brother Dean had passed away and we were needed in Florida to attend the memorial service to be held in Dean's honor. We packed our belongings, said our goodbyes and left the Rockies on a high speed run across the country.

Dean is one of the most unforgettable people I have ever met. He was totally outgoing and could start up some revelry with perfect strangers. One time he had visited Debbie and I at home and we went into town for dinner. Dean had a group of people standing in the middle of the sidewalk and singing together before I even had a chance to complete parking the car. We walked with him on a trail to a local waterfall and Dean initiated deep conversations with everyone we passed. He spoke of family and love and the excitement of living. It was shameful that he had been forced to endure the breakup from and subsequent knife attack by his ex-wife. It was unfortunate that Dean began to rely on the bottle to salve his depression and had been unable to get his nose from being buried in that bottle constantly. The doctor said it was the alcohol that consumed and killed him; we knew it was the broken heart that took him from this earth.

The Clark family gathered along with Dean's three grown children to honor his memory. We all had tales to tell of Dean's large spirit. It had been Dean's desire to have his ashes placed in the ocean. After a short service we drove to the nearest beach and Dean's mother, children and siblings walked waist deep into the water still wearing their church clothes and carrying helium balloons. Debbie was too unbalanced to walk safely into the water and I stood with her letting the surf beat up against our ankles as Debbie's mother herself released the remains of her eldest child into the warm waters of the Gulf of Mexico. There were very few tears that day. No one present had been surprised at Dean's early demise. We were all just saddened at his defeat and remembered him kindly.

We remained in Florida with Debbie's mom a few extra days to make sure she was well and could adjust. Debbie's mom has always been a pillar of strength and calm and this occasion was no different. We started back on the highway heading home with just one more place to stop.

We had reconnected with Dean's children and they had requested we stop at their home in Jacksonville and we were glad to agree and to strengthen the family bond. Brooke, Amber and Cory had all grown to be beautiful and responsible adults. Brooke and Amber had become nurses. Cory was attending school. We were so proud of them. The day before we left for their house Amber called us and asked if we would care to attend a comedy club performance by a fellow named Tommy Chong. Amber went on to explain he had been a member of the Cheech & Chong comedy duo and I played along as if I had never heard of him. I kept asking her why she thought her Aunt Debbie and I would appreciate such humor. We had a great night out and have now made Jacksonville a stopping place on our yearly Christmas visits to Debbie's mom.

Debbie and I returned home to the newest version of our life. We could continue to make it as long as we continued to scale back on the activities we loved to engage in. Our walking was necessary for our mental well-being as well as being an integral part of Debbie's physical therapy. Each day's outing made Debbie a little bit stronger and once again we were measuring her progress by how far she could go on any given path.

We still enjoyed music. At home we listen to an extremely wide variety of different artists. Anything from the Allman Brothers to Frank Zappa. We were listening to more jazz than ever before and were becoming interested in the history of this uniquely American form of music. We became aware of musical giants like Thelonius Monk, Sonny Rollins and Art Blakey, Miles Davis and John Coltrane. We had always known the names but now we could begin to identify the music.

Living where we do in the Blue Ridge Mountains it would be impossible to avoid bluegrass. Debbie and I had been attending the Merlefest festival hosted every year by our fellow county resident, Doc Watson. In fact, Merlefests were some of the few occasions (other than Grateful Dead concerts) that Debbie and I would meet in those years prior to our marriage. This festival honors the memory of Doc's son, Merle, who had been killed in a farm tractor accident. Many of the best musicians from around the world performed there and Debbie and I were both fans.

It was no longer feasible for Debbie to go to such events. The walking involved and the distance to the nearest Port-a-Jon became overwhelming obstacles to us. I still wished her to take part in whatever she could though and we scaled back our concert going just as we had been forced to scale back our walking. The cost of concerts also had become an issue for us now that we were on a limited income.

One night I did take Debbie to see Doc Watson and Sam Bush (an incredible mandolin player) performing at the auditorium on the campus of Appalachian State University in nearby Boone. I figured that since this would be a theater environment with seating for all that Debbie would be able to enjoy the show. We arrived early to allow Debbie sufficient time to use the rest room and to find our seats. Everything went really well until the intermission. The folks who had been sitting to Debbie's left were a white haired elderly couple and when they stood up to go to the lobby Debbie, being the polite and courteous person that she is, also stood up to allow them to pass. Debbie stood there, and the couple stood there too. It was a stalemate for several moments until I recognized the problem. Debbie had used the seat in front of her to pull herself up from her chair and she was still clinging to it with all her might preventing the folks from getting by. I apologized sheepishly and asked Debbie to move her hands. She didn't understand why the people were still standing there and she couldn't figure why I was asking her to move. Finally, I lifted Debbie's hands and the couple went on. Debbie never did understand how she was blocking their way and when they returned to their seats they came from the opposite aisle.

A new activity did begin for Debbie in the late summer. She was deemed eligible to take part in a therapeutic horseback riding program run by volunteers out of the Blowing Rock stables. The program is called Blazing Saddles and allows children and adults who are handicapped to learn to care for and groom horses. They are then helped into the saddle and are protected by several volunteers each who maintain safety positions alongside the horse. Debbie had always enjoyed horses and had done some riding in her past. I did not believe that they would succeed in getting Debbie into the saddle. But they did.

It took three people to assist Debbie up the steps of the mounting block and to swing her legs into the stirrups. Once Debbie was sitting erect in the saddle the horse did all the rest of the work. I was so glad for Debbie that she had been able to sit on this lofty perch on the horse's back, that I once more cried at one of her accomplishments.

Debbie was taught the command to make the horse go forward and was taught that she could direct the horse with the reins and by squeezing her legs against the horse's side. The volunteers who stood guard and maintained a handhold on the lead ensured her safety. The horse's name was Dude and we had great fun repeating the word Dude stretching out the vowel sound as long as we could. "Duuuuuuuuude!" We have come to look forward to spring and Debbie's reuniting with Dude. Unfortunately the program has been suffering because of a lack of funds and we do not know if it will be able to continue. I hope they can, as the joy brought to the riders is immeasurable. Debbie so looks forward to the hour a week she spends with the horses. Dude, Callie and Shrek have become her friends.

On Election Day Debbie and I voted proudly for President Barack Obama. We were thrilled with his proposals to provide universal health care for all citizens as we had seen first hand how little insurance companies cared for the people their policies insured. More than once we had to have our doctors fight for treatments that we knew would be beneficial to Debbie's health and that the insurance companies had denied. We were also not unaware of the message that the election of a non-white would send to the world and to the children of our own country. Americans, at heart, want to live in peace and this election proved to the world that we meant that. In addition, the election proved once and for all that America is the land of freedom and opportunity and that any child could grow up to be President.

Our dreams were not quite as lofty. We would be satisfied to just survive and have Debbie become more balanced and adept in her walking. As the New Year of 2009 began Debbie and I joined with our countrymen in experiencing a rebirth of hope.

CHAPTER 30

Debbie and I had settled into what has become our daily routine. Debbie now sleeps for 12-15 hours a day and leaves me to cope with the silence of the long mornings on my own. Her communication and conversational skills have dissipated to the point where I must work extremely hard to elicit anything other than a "yeah, right or good" response. Debbie has come to make daily choices that I believe are harmful to her long-term prospects. She refuses my many entreaties to engage in exercise or to take a short walk. Debbie refuses to build upon the strength that engaging in activity affords her. We have noticed that if Debbie walks for several days in a row her stride does lengthen and her overall gait is stronger. Conversely we have also become aware that if Debbie does not engage in activity then the next time she does she must relearn the stride she had worked so hard to achieve. Practice and repetition have become a requirement and unfortunately Debbie has learned how to repeat the usage of the word "No" more frequently than she should.

This seeming lack of effort on her part coupled with the monotone of her speech and the incredible lack of emotional response has brought me to the brink of desperation. The tedium of our routine has drowned me in depression. I am so lonely that on some days I actually welcome the call of a credit card offer just so that I can speak to someone. I have clearly crossed a line that leads to insanity. It is difficult when the options of your life have become so limited that you really just don't have any choices left at all. Yes, I could leave the house and go out, but then Debbie would be unattended and I could not bear the thought of her injuring herself and my not being there to help. So, in effect my daily options are now, I can stay or I can stay. Nice choice, I think to myself. I invariably choose to stay.

Occasionally Debbie did step up and we would have a wonderful day having a picnic in the forest just like in our past. These days were like a fresh breeze blowing my troubles away. I recognized that there was still a part of me that could appreciate the beauty of my environment and that there could still be joy in our existence. I was just struggling to hold that feeling and was not able to make the few hours a week where Debbie was interacting appropriately compensate for all the huge hunks of time I was spending totally alone.

My emotions had become worn thin and were always on the surface. A ray of sunlight filtering its way through the green canopy of the forest could bring me to tears of joy. Debbie's refusal to follow my lead and direction while attempting to surmount an obstacle such as a fallen log would wrench my back leaving me crying tears of pain and anger. I had learned to cry at just about anything. A snatch of music, the sight of a deer, the buzz of the hummingbird, the passing of a cloud all would elicit the melancholy I was now constantly surrounded by.

We were struck by a terrible blow in mid-August. Our companion and friend, D.D. the Dog, stumbled while walking a flat trail with us one day. She froze and fell just as her mistress Debbie had many times previously. D.D. did find her way back up and followed us as we returned to the car. We just assumed she had picked up a thorn in her paw, as she exhibited no further symptoms for a couple days. Then the dog fell again. I took her to the veterinarian who said that D.D. had some form of neurological illness that could be a brain tumor. I freaked out and said that could not be as the coincidences were too much to bear. I explained to the vet that Debbie was the victim of a brain tumor and he then understood my reaction. The vet explained that we could send D.D. to the "doggie neurologist" where a diagnosis could be obtained following an exam and a MRI scan. The vet further explained that this workup would cost several thousand dollars and would still not have addressed any treatment options for the dog. We could not afford such an expense and it was decided to place the dog on steroids and hope for the best.

The next three weeks D.D. would lie on the couch and I would carry food and water to her. We knew something was drastically wrong with her when she would refuse to eat from a canned tin of beef. Some days the steroids would allow D.D. to act strong and she would still bravely lift herself and join us when we went for a ride in the car and would attempt to follow along just as she always had. Only now D.D. was unable to keep up with Debbie and would just sit in the middle of the trail and I would have to pick her up and carry her back to the car. Each afternoon and every morning Debbie and I would talk about whether or when we would take D.D. to be put down. We were distraught and I was getting by on nothing but inertia. I continued moving because I could not stop. On some days I had to lift both Debbie and our dog from the ground after a fall. It was too much.

D.D. passed away quietly one morning at the foot of Debbie's bed. We buried her in our front yard in a spot in full view of our living room window. I miss that dog and will till the day I die.

D.D.'s demise led Debbie to a major self-discovery. Debbie had been on anti-depressive medications for several years and she requested that she stop taking them. I asked her why and she said it was because she could not feel anything at D.D.'s loss. She knew she was sad, we both loved that dog, but she couldn't feel her sadness and she wanted to. I called the doctor who directed me how to safely have Debbie step down from the medication. This was a positive step for Debbie and symbolized to me a regeneration of her spirit. I would like to say that Debbie's personality snapped back to the buoyancy of her past days, it didn't. Debbie has, however, become more able to hear the urgency in my requests for her to remain active and she also became able to recognize my plea for more coherent interactions with her.

We traveled little this year. Debbie's shakiness when walking had forced us to curtail almost all activity other than walking on wide flat trails or on paved sidewalks. We began to appear frequently at the local park. Several times a week I would escort Debbie on the paved path that circled the park. We could take a short loop of ¼ mile or could extend that walk to ½ or ¾ of a mile if Debbie was feeling strong and if the weather was agreeable.

Debbie would say hello to each and every person we passed. We walked so slowly that frequently we would pass the same person several times as we made our single circuit around. Many of the people we met were extremely friendly to us and we began to recognize many of our neighbors as our appearances in the park became more frequent. Many people would comment on Debbie's walking stick and ask if Debbie had made it. She would truthfully answer that only God can make a tree. Debbie is totally unable to involve in dissembling. She speaks only the truth as she sees it with no exaggeration or desire to confuse or tease. Debbie now speaks in completely literal fashion and sometimes the use of idioms will get her to correct or question someone. For Debbie it is no longer as hot as Hades, it is precisely ninety-one degrees.

One day while strolling Debbie said hello to a well-dressed woman in her sixties. The second time we passed her Debbie said hello again and this time the woman responded with a hello of her own. The third time we passed, the woman stayed to talk with us. We explained that we lived nearby and used the park frequently to allow Debbie the exercise she required. The woman went on and remarked how friendly we were and then exclaimed, "How wonderful it is to share the park with you wonderful people. And how fabulous it is that we are all Christians". I bit my tongue. I so wanted to lift this person from her disillusionment. It was nice to be considered friendly enough that I could be taken for a Christian, but friendly or not, I am still a Jew. This woman's attitude crystallized for me what is wrong with our country. People just naturally assume that the only "good" or "friendly" people come in the same variety as themselves. This is completely false. Good people come in all colors, shapes and creeds. This Christian woman probably did not mean us any harm and more than likely did wish and pray for Debbie's health as she had said she would. Would she have done so knowing of my Jewish upbringing? Would she have done so knowing that Debbie considered herself a pagan? The three of us all share belief in a greater power, and more importantly all share the same time and space on this earth. Shouldn't that fact alone be enough for us to find a common ground? Must we, as she was so obviously insisting, call our deity by the same name? I propose that Debbie and I in our mixed marriage of different religious upbringings demonstrate more true "Christian" values than this woman is possibly capable of.

Debbie earned a new nickname that fall. Debbie was comfortably in her easy chair watching the television and she settled on a telecast of the New York City marathon. The announcer kept referring to an American runner named Meb Keflezghi who had taken the lead in the race. Now I have always enjoyed watching televised sports. I mostly prefer the team sports of baseball and football but am familiar with all of them. I had gotten into the habit of repeating an athlete's name and asking Debbie rhetorically, "Who is this guy? Where do we get guys like that?" I jumped right upon Meb's name. "Who is Meb Keflezghi and why do we have guys like that?" Of course I am just joking around and trying to elicit a smile or a laugh from Debbie but Debbie always responds with no humor at all. "He's a runner from the United States." After the conclusion of the long race that Keflezghi had been able to win I began calling Debbie Meb Keflezghi. It was partly the rhyming similarity between Deb and Meb and partly the way the sound of the name Meb Keflezghi just rolled off my tongue. It was mostly the way that Debbie responded to my calling her Meb Keflezghi that sealed the deal. She accepted that she and he had things in common. They were both running marathons and were both in it to win.

I have since researched Meb's web page and I now quote him, "Life is like a marathon. Stick to your dreams and don't ever give up." Meb and Debbie have much in common. I wish further success to Meb Keflezghi, the real one, and thank him for the inspiration his victory in New York brought to Debbie. Keep going Meb Keflezghi, both of you!

We did have to endure one very disturbing episode. One afternoon Katherine, Debbie's physical therapist, informed us that we would need to drop Debbie from the physical therapy rolls. It seems the hospital was not going to be reimbursed for Debbie's visits. She had outstayed her Medicare welcome. The thought of winter coming along with the realization that the weather would naturally curtail Debbie's outdoor exercising made the prospect of no scheduled physical therapy appointments even more distressing. I called Dr. Desjardins and she maintained that Debbie should have and needed to continue her therapy. It had always been my understanding that if the doctor prescribed it then the hospital would follow through. In addition, payment was not an issue as I had worked closely with a financial officer to ensure that Debbie's accounts would be settled by a government grant in addition to Medicare. Again, before I continue, let me remind you that Debbie and I had paid our premiums for a lifetime and were entitled to the payout on our claims.

In either case Katherine's hands were tied and her supervisor would not allow Debbie to placed on the schedule. Katherine set up an appointment for me with her supervisor. I will not divulge the supervisor's name to protect her identity but honestly she is deserving of nothing from me.

I sat in the administrator's office and the supervisor sat behind a large desk across from me. The administrator told me she must remove Debbie from the schedule and I reminded her of the obligation to provide the services that had been legally prescribed by a physician. I reminded her that she is not a doctor and could not make a medical decision such as removing a patient from care. She then told me she had spoken personally with Debbie's doctor and was following the physician's orders. I was taken aback as my earlier conversation with Dr. Desjardins had not gone that way.

I asked again, "Did you speak with Debbie's doctor?"

The reply was, "Yes, I did."

"OK, then", I questioned. "What did the doctor say?"

"Well, he said that Debbie needed to be removed for a four month period."

"He said that?"

"Yes."

"And you personally spoke with the doctor?" I knew I had caught this person in a blatant lie. After hearing another affirmative response I snapped the trap shut on this woman who had the audacity to lie directly to my face.

"Debbie's doctor is a woman, not a man, and you never in your life spoke with her. You are a liar."

I wish I could say that this solved the matter. It didn't and Debbie's name was purged from the therapy schedule. I wrote a complaining letter to the hospital administration but to my knowledge nothing has come of it. Perhaps the lying woman was reprimanded privately. I do not know.

As the year came to its conclusion the realization hit me that I had not spent an evening away from Debbie in nearly two years. Debbie and I had used to attend a yearly event in Asheville called the Christmas Jam. The event is hosted by local musician, Warren Haynes, and benefits Habitat for Humanity. We used to join with our friends Broc and Michelle and would party into the wee hours of the morning, as the long list of visiting musicians would continue to play until 4 or 5 A.M. Broc asked if I would join them this year. I arranged for my brother-in-law Brad to stay with Debbie and I took the night off. It was a very different thing for me to be out of the house on my own. The music touched me and I remembered once more that there is still a joie de vivre of my own that I was sublimating in my sacrifice of caring for Debbie full-time. After the concert and a few hours sleep I returned home, thanking Broc for his thoughts of me, and returning once again to the drudgery of my daily routine.

I still loved Debbie and I was determined to remain at her side as she faced the future. I could not, however, state with complete sincerity that I didn't wish for a more normal existence.

CHAPTER 31

The winters of the Blue Ridge Mountains can be severe. We are not southern enough so as to have no winter and the elevation that cools us in the summer continues to cool us in the winter. Our little corner of the world is usually 7-10 degrees cooler than the surrounding flatlands. This means if it is 35 degrees and raining in the Piedmont (the flatland plain east of the Blue Ridge), it is 25 degrees and snowing where we live. This had never been an issue for us in the past but now with Debbie's imbalance ice and snow have become a sentence of quarantine. We are locked in our house and unable to travel at all. I can get free to perform necessary grocery expeditions but Debbie cannot go outdoors safely.

My niece Jennifer and her boyfriend Aaron had joined my nephew Adam in Tucson. Adam suggested we come spend some time with him to escape from the harshness that winter was besieging us with. We accepted his invitation and began travel westward the first week of February when Dr. Desjardins had cleared Debbie.

We made a stop at Carlsbad Caverns that clearly demonstrated Debbie's continuing loss of strength. Debbie was unable to complete a circuit of the Big Room and had to be assisted on a wheelchair brought by a park ranger. This was a disappointing beginning to our trip and made it abundantly clear to me that Debbie's activities would have to be closely monitored.

Two days after our arrival in Tucson our vehicle broke down. This was disastrous as the resultant repairs ran $1800 and Debbie and I had to reach into our savings in order to settle the bill and become mobile again.

The rest of the trip went smoothly. We limited Debbie's walks to a half mile or less but were still able to discover wonderful places to rest and enjoy our picnic lunches. We stayed four weeks with Adam. He is a kind and giving spirit and along with some help from Jennifer I was also able to getaway on some mornings for some longer expeditions on my own. I was thrilled to discover some waterfalls in the desert and marveled at the sight of torrents of water falling down huge cliff faces surrounded by Saguaro cactus. The southwest is a beautiful part of our country, even more so when enjoyed in the wintertime.

We could not leave the west without stopping to see Mike and Debbie in Colorado Springs. They have been marvelous friends throughout the years and it is just so comfortable for us to spend time with them. This trip they had arranged for us to spend a weekend at the Ojo Caliente hot spring spa and resort located in northern New Mexico. They treated Debbie to an aromatherapy spa treatment. Debbie was wrapped in warm towels infused with sage. She received a massage and a shampoo using sage oils. This was a special treat that our limited budget would never have allowed and demonstrates the graciousness of our friends.

Debbie did have one issue with me there. The four of us walked over together to take a hot soak. Debbie insisted that she wear her clothing rather than a bathrobe, as the rest of us were about to do. I could not dissuade her. I told her I would await her at the entrance to the ladies locker room and stood in the cold wearing nothing but a bathing suit and a bathrobe. I began shivering as my wait grew longer and longer. Finally Debbie emerged. My teeth were chattering by now and I didn't just want a hot soaking bath. I needed one to halt the spread of frostbite. We enjoyed our time in the hot springs and when it was time to return to our cabin I urged Debbie to hurry, as I did not want to grow cold again. I waited and waited. The heat that had built up because of my immersion in the hot water was quickly fading away and I grew cold once more. This time Debbie emerged from the locker room wearing a bathrobe and nothing else. She had no pants! Debbie had forgotten which locker she placed her belongings in. Of course the staff was able to search all the lockers and find Debbie's clothing later that evening but I have continued to utilize this incident every time that Debbie fails to follow my advice and insists on doing things her way. I remind her of the time she had no pants.

We returned home the first day of April to a marvelous Blue Ridge spring. Our first order of business was to re-enroll Debbie in physical therapy. The Medicare requirement of a break in therapy appointments had been satisfied but I did not wish to have Debbie return to her previous program because I was still annoyed by the woman who had lied to me. I saw no reason that her program should benefit by Debbie's return. I called all the other therapy providers in town and they all suggested that because of Debbie's condition she should see Katherine, the best trained therapist in our area for patients with Debbie's needs. I sucked up my pride and had Debbie placed back on the schedule. We have been attending sessions throughout the remainder of the year. Katherine and all the other staff and therapists were glad to see Debbie and have been nothing but friendly. The lying supervisor, however, continues to work and despite walking right past us numerous times as we wait for Debbie's appointment to begin has never acknowledged our presence at all. All she need do would be to apologize for having told me a blatant lie. This person has been unable to do so and try as I might her failure to apologize has made it difficult for me to forgive her.

Debbie and I, and all our friends for that matter, had always been on the periphery of American politics. We voted for the candidates throughout the years that supported humanitarian instead of corporate values but never really felt connected to the process. This changed in 2010 when our friend Billy chose to become involved and earned the Democratic nomination to run for the United States Congress. We were thrilled to have some one we knew and could trust to seek this office and offered our services to the campaign.

I spent many hours assisting in the collation of names we could draw upon for financial support. Being an independent democrat Billy did not receive over three quarters of a million dollars in big oil money the way his opponent did. Debbie and I also donned our Billy for Congress t-shirts and actively campaigned and made public appearances at local events urging our neighbors to support Billy in his efforts to provide health care for all while still maintaining a balanced budget. Democrats have been the only party to present a balanced budget in my lifetime. President Clinton left office with a budget surplus, which the excesses and failure of the Bush administration turned into the largest budget deficit of our lifetime. I spoke with many people throughout the election season and could not understand the logic of anyone who insisted they were voting Republican. I could sense hostility targeted toward President Obama mostly due to his race. I was saddened. What I found even more disturbing was the apathy of the younger voters in our district. The college students did not turn out to vote. Only 8% of the voting age students cared enough to appear at the ballot box. They will be paying the price of their inaction quickly as loans for college tuition are on the GOP hit list. Needless to say, Billy lost. I have never been so proud of a friend before. I did not know how Billy was able to face the evil that now pervades our country without losing his temper a single time. He always calmly explained the differences between the goals of the two parties. All we have been saying is that the needs of our citizens are worthier than the wants of multi-national corporations that steal from government coffers frequently and still manage to lay off and fire our workers while shipping jobs to foreign countries in search of cheaper labor. Our district, along with the rest of the country refused to hear. It will cost us.

We are now also without a pet for the first time in our married life. Our aged cat, C.C., had to be put down. She was nineteen years old and no longer had the ability to lift herself and walk. We had watched hopelessly as she had continued to decline and contented ourselves with the fact that she was in no apparent pain. We cried together as the cat was injected and then was laid in Debbie's lap while it breathed its last. For several nights afterward I would have sworn the cat was still in the house and I saw her figure walking through our hallway. I have since overcome my fear and have relearned how to set mousetraps.

There have been no major health issues for Debbie to confront this year. Her condition has seemingly stabilized. MRI scans continue to be taken twice a year to ensure that no threat has been posed by the activity inside Debbie's brain. She has survived and endured the nine years after her tumor and her brain surgery.

Debbie and I have settled into our life with cancer. Sometimes the sheer boredom of the hours I spend waiting overwhelm me and I shed a few tears. Mostly I just continue on as best I can. And so does Debbie.

CHAPTER 32

You may have gotten the impression from reading this account that I am some kind of hero or saint. Nothing could be further from the truth. It is true that I have remained loyal to Debbie and have honored the marriage vow of staying through sickness and in health. Others may not have, but my love for Debbie remains unabated and so I stay and try to make each day a loving experience for us both. Sometimes I succeed. Sometimes I have failed miserably.

I have become a lonely person as the years have progressed. We are unable to take part in many of the social activities and gatherings we used to attend so frequently. We spend almost all our time by ourselves and as you have seen Debbie's depth of conversation does lack some sparkle these days. I long for companionship. I have accepted my role as full-time caregiver and will maintain it, as I know that the way in that I care for Debbie will be the defining moments of my lifetime. I pray for the patience I will need to assist Debbie in her journey. I confess that patience has not always been my best virtue.

I have lost my temper on a number of occasions in the last several years. My frustration at Debbie's inability to follow through on her promises to maintain her exercise regimen, her insistence on her own logic that defies the normal rules of physics and the endless tension of waiting to see when or if she will arise in the mornings have taken serious tolls on my emotional reserves. The repetition thousands of times of the same safety rules I have been forced to impose have taken their toll and I cannot go through the same thing again. Sometimes I just explode.

I no longer have full control of myself. The buttons are pushed and I go off like a rocket into a loud and prolonged tirade of ranting and profanity. I am ashamed of myself. And I am sorry.

I am just a man being faced directly with the slow and steady decline of his beautiful wife who was stricken with a life threatening illness just when our life as a happily married couple was beginning to find its stride. All has been taken from us. We have become marginal people and our very existence has become a political football for politicians who value the campaign contributions they receive more than the lives of the constituents they represent. Debbie would have died several times had her doctors and I not fought on her behalf.

I say that Debbie's life, even though it has become a damaged one, still has value. I see that in the smile of a young girl we met at a Doc Watson performance this past summer who accepted a handmade red, white and blue bead necklace that she had admired and that Debbie took off her neck and gave to her. I see it in the joy of our neighbors in the park who are delighted that Debbie still struggles to maintain her stamina and that she has accepted her fate stoically. I see it in the words of my own mother who following her own stroke said that Debbie has been her inspiration. I see it in the faces of the newer patients who appear at the Brain Tumor Clinic and are afraid as they see their lives changing but who take comfort in the fact of Debbie's continued survival.

Our life on this earth is tenuous and precarious. We owe it to each other to care and provide for those who are no longer able. Nothing we accomplish is worth anything if it comes at the expense of the weak. We are stronger than that and we are better human beings than that.

Debbie is!

The Tenth Year

Jeff Block

CHAPTER 1

It's been a year since I last sat to write about life with Debbie. Yes, we have survived it and I expect to continue for as long as I may. Last year upon the release of Nine Years After I didn't realize the impact it's writing would have upon me. I have laid my soul bare and spoken of intimacies that perhaps I should not have. I have offered opinions that may have been found offensive. Most importantly I had set out goals that I intended to live by.

I promised, publicly and in writing, that I would strive to make every day of our lives together as fun and enjoyable as I possibly could. I have been procrastinating in fear of this moment. I have not wished to face the events of the past year.

I can begin here as I did previously by telling you that my mornings are still the worst. The hateful pressure of silence while Debbie sleeps away her mornings and early afternoons has me tense by the time Debbie awakes. The mind numbing routine of providing for Debbie's safety and comfort has caused my depressions to find me crying almost daily. My tantrums have reached epic and embarrassing proportions. I feel as I am a total failure all of the time. In this past year I have become responsible, in Debbie's eyes, for the failure of some movies to please her (after all, what was I thinking when I ordered that one?), for cooking sausage patties which she loves, in the same way for the last ten years (according to Debbie now they're burned), for being lucky enough to have flat tires on consecutive days (even though they were both brand new and the service center replaced them) and just generally not having the extra arms necessary to perform all of Debbie's chores an hour or two before she thinks of them.

Debbie so rarely appears in our house anymore. There is an alternate personality residing in her body that has seized control of her actions for much of every day. She is not or never has been a schizophrenic, yet the brain damage she has suffered over time has altered her and for the most part she is unaware of this. When I ask for her patience and indulgence she reverts to her sweet self and we momentarily reconnect. Unfortunately the reconnections do not linger.

I have teasingly been calling myself the staff at the "tin roof inn"- our home in the mountains where the rain does rattle on the roof during storms. I tell Debbie that the staff is sorry for her discomfort and that her day's stay will be offered as a complimentary gift in hope that she will continue to let "us" serve her. In a voice I can barely hear she says, "Thanks very much". I continue going about the chores of domesticity, cooking and cleaning, and Debbie remains in position glued to the television screen. The pure truth of the matter is that I miss Debbie. I miss her spirit and exuberance. It hurts me to my core to watch her struggle with her steps and I am shaken each time I must help her up from the ground.

Two thousand eleven, the tenth year since Debbie's diagnosis as a brain cancer patient has been another year of roller coaster riding. Most of our days have been uneventful, calm and serene. We still take short walks and enjoy the flowing of the river at our local park. We occasionally have a picnic lunch at an outdoor overlook and still host those willing to spend a day or three visiting with us and the beautiful Blue Ridge. Debbie still proclaims her love for me and on the most rare of occasions will offer genuine thanks for the care she receives from me. I invariably cry when Debbie speaks to me with sincerity. So, am I a failure or not? The year has passed and Debbie still wishes to stay here with me but I have also embarrassed myself in ways I may never recover from. You've come so far with us, read on, see what you think.

CHAPTER 2

"What?" I ask Debbie as I carry her dinner to her.

"What?" is her response.

And I, in my perversity, inquire once more with, "What?"

We will repeat the word "what" several more times and with each repetition you can feel Debbie's frustration level rise until she finally catches the twinkles in the inflections of my voice. Her face lights up, she smiles the crooked smile where her eyes get wide and the right side of her mouth lifts in a grin.

"That's not wat", she says, "that's chicken!"

"Right!" I say and she repeats my word but the joke has been completed and her responsive "right" has been stated in a quiet monotone while her smile has disappeared. I had Debbie there for a moment but she is lost again.

I have always enjoyed telling and sharing jokes. To my everlasting shame, and as you have already surmised, I like puns. I realize this is not an endearing character trait but in honesty I must claim it. I have also always said that a joke isn't funny if it has to be explained, but I am going to explain the origin of the "wat" joke because it is still funny for Debbie and I and we really don't have much to laugh about these days.

Back when I lived in Georgia teaching school in the early 90's I used to travel frequently to Atlanta where I took the opportunity to eat in an Ethiopian restaurant. The ambience of such an exotic cuisine is quite different. There is no silverware in sight at your table. The food is served on thick, spongy sourdough bread and the various types of stew are placed atop the bread that is called injera. You wrap the stew in the injera and eat with your fingers. You are encouraged, if you are lovers, to feed each other. It is a unique style of eating and is quite fun. The stews, which may be made from lamb, goat, beef or various vegetables, are called wat. Lamb wat, beef wat, vegetable wat. Being the punny guy that I am I could not resist the temptation of coining the phrase, "Wat's for dinner?" The correct response when eating Ethiopian is of course to respond, "Right!" Debbie and I have sought out Ethiopian restaurants during our travels and I am sure that the joy we made for ourselves with our word play silliness added immensely to our enjoyment of those evenings.

Debbie enjoys the word play. She is a fan of the Abbott & Costello comedy team and the skit they have made famous concerning the names of the players on the local baseball team is guaranteed to make her laugh. We have altered that routine slightly to accommodate current events. I am always happy to be Debbie's straight man.

I ask, "Debbie, who is the president of China?"

Debbie gleefully responds, "Right!"

I play to our audience and ask once more, "Do you know who is the president of China?"

"Exactly!" Debbie looks like the cat that swallowed the canary. She can barely control herself and it is such a pleasure to see her playful side again.

"What is the name of the man that is president of China?"

Debbie answers, "Who."

I act annoyed with her, "The man who is president of China, that's who!"

"Right!" And we can continue on with this zaniness until our audience (victims?) finally figure out that the president of China is a man named Hu. It's OK if you groan, I know it's a bad pun, Debbie might know, but we don't care.

The repetition of the word "what" now allows me to jar Debbie's memory and to elicit a smile from her. I so wish to be able to continue our conversation and when Debbie is willing we will engage in further word play.

Sometimes we come upon a roadblock and Debbie's mind just hits a wall. One evening we began with the "whats" and then branched out to other meanings of the word "what". Now, of course having begun with the acceptance of wat being phonetically equal to what, we had to include all possible homonyms of the word "what". So, one night we spoke of the electrical term identified as a watt. We researched basic electrical physics and discovered and relearned the definitions of watt, volt, ampere and ohms. One night we discussed the inventor James Watt and that naturally led to discussing the inventors of the telephone and of the incandescent light bulb. Debbie remembered Alexander Graham Bell whose name so sounds like the name of the inventor of the telephone should sound. That reminded me of Thomas Crapper whose name destined him to become the inventor of the flush toilet. (No shit, you can look it up!) But then after a few chuckles, Debbie's mind went dark. There was no longer a light on in her attic. She could not for the life of her recall the name of the man who invented the light bulb. I have learned that it is better to let Debbie search her mind rather than let her take the easy way out and just tell her. She will insist I tell her, she will get angry and her voice will rise from its usual monotone. "Tell me!" she demands. I have, however, seen the sense of accomplishment she feels when she finally comes up with a correct answer to something. You may remember the time she chased down a doctor to answer an arithmetic question he had posed. This time it was poor Thomas Edison who had escaped from Debbie's remembrance of history.

I gave a prompt. "He also invented the phonograph".

"Right!" I gave the hand signal upon hearing Debbie use the word right and to acknowledge that she had said it with feeling. Debbie went on.

"Yes, and we visited his winter home in Florida with my mother".

That was correct. One Christmas while visiting Deb's mom we took a day trip and visited Edison's winter quarters in Naples, Florida. There was a large and priceless collection of Edison's phonographs there and Debbie went on to describe the megaphone appearance of their speakers. She remembered the old cars parked in the garage and even remembered that the adjoining estate belonged to automobile giant, Henry Ford. She still couldn't remember Edison's name. We went to sleep that night and Debbie had not achieved illumination.

The next day we continued to plumb the depths of Debbie's memory. I would have been satisfied with the shallow response of Edison's name but Debbie went deeper.

"Yes", Debbie asked, "do you remember the time we were in New Jersey staying with your sister and went to the laboratory where we saw his library and the tiny movie studio out in the parking lot?"

Again Debbie was correct. We had visited Edison's factory and laboratory in New Jersey. We saw his library. Debbie even mentioned the time we watched an episode of The Simpsons set in that very library. The tiny movie studio outback had actually been used in the production of some of the first ever movie features. Many people forget that Edison was also instrumental in the development of the moving picture camera. Debbie hadn't forgotten, but she still just couldn't remember his name! This went on for months. Every now and again I would ask Debbie the name of the man who invented the light bulb. One morning when we hadn't even brought it up for a couple weeks Debbie blurted out, "Thomas Edison!"

Debbie forgets many more things these days. Edison's name, while historically important, is not a matter of life and limb. The rules I have established for her safety are. Many are the times Debbie has found herself looking up at the world from the ground because she has forgotten a safety precept I have repeated with her thousands of times. "Ask for help, stay away from corners, don't try to walk and carry things at the same time, don't stand near the steps, lift your feet- don't drag them." These phrases repeated literally thousands of times- Debbie is unable to remember them. It is sad for her and frustrating and aggravating for me.

Usually Debbie can tell you the correct day and date, just not always. She is almost always within a month of the correct date. Her calendar approximations really do force me to address the question of where does the time go?

Debbie also cannot remember the logistical details of her schedule. I daily remind her of when her and/or our next appointment is. Physical therapy on Tuesday at 3 P.M., visiting a friend on Saturday. She is always confused now when awakening. I may have told her fifty times or more when her next MRI is scheduled. Comes that day, she has forgotten.

"Is that today?"

Sometimes I respond hastily and harshly that it is. Sometimes I do better and respond with an inquisitive and robust, "What?"

And we continue.

CHAPTER 3

We spent Christmas at home. This was a unique event for us as we had almost always gone to Debbie's mom's house for the holidays. We exchanged small trinkets. Debbie presented me with one of her handmade cards.

I knew we would be spending an extended period of time in Florida over the winter and so with Virginia's complete understanding we remained at home until after Debbie's appointment at the Brain Tumor Clinic the first week of February.

It was cold. The Blue Ridge had fallen into a deep freeze; the lakes and ponds were suitable for skating. We did not go out often. Temperatures were hovering near zero and the ice in our driveway never had a chance to melt. Our car would not go up our slick and icy driveway. I could walk to the bottom of the drive where I kept the car safely parked, but Debbie could not. I was forced to call for assistance from friends every time Debbie needed to be somewhere. In retrospect January was the calmest month we would experience until summertime.

After a clean evaluation by Dr. Desjardins at Duke we continued on from Durham to Florida where we settled in with Debbie's mother for what we hoped would be a calm, peaceful and warm six week stay. It was warm. In fact, the weather was just about perfect with sunny days and temperatures in the low 80's. Our stay, unfortunately, was neither peaceful nor calm and I'm afraid that was largely my fault. I had hoped for help from Debbie's mother and although Virginia was quite willing and wanting to help, she and I just did not agree on what was now necessary for Debbie's safety.

Just past a week into our stay Debbie awoke one afternoon and announced that she wanted to take a shower. I asked her to wait five minutes while I gathered my own toiletries and got undressed. It was my intention, as I had been doing at home for months, to stand alongside Debbie in the shower to help her maintain her balance in the wet environment of the shower stall. Virginia asked why I just did not let Debbie have her independence and let her shower herself. Virginia pointed out that her shower was a walk-in variety and that Debbie would not have to step over a tub. That was all Debbie needed to hear. She was inside the bathroom and in the stall before I had a chance to undress. Debbie was also lying crumpled in a corner of the stall, crying and with a bump on the back of her head by the time I had gotten undressed. Accidents, as I have learned over the years, happen in the blink of an eye. Of course, Virginia came running for me as soon as Debbie hit the wet tiled floor.

I helped Debbie up and placed her head under the nozzle to wash off the blood. There was going to be a bump, but Debbie seemed fine. She knew where she was; she knew what day it was and even knew we were scheduled to visit her sister for a barbeque. She seemed capable of maintaining her balance and we continued with the day's plans. Several hours passed until later that evening Debbie complained of exhaustion, asked to lie down and promptly vomited all over the bedding. She was unable to stand or support her weight. It was all I could do to drag her by her shoulders with her feet dangling uselessly as I brought her to the commode. We called an ambulance for the first time since Debbie's initial presentation of a seizure had begun this nightmare ten years ago.

I could sense the hostility of the doctor in the emergency room. He was unhappy to be treating a Medicaid patient and made it clear with his tone that he was not satisfied with our insurance arrangements. He did authorize a CAT scan but would offer no opinion as to what had happened to cause Debbie, who had walked with me the day before for a mile through the palms and saw palmettos of a local park, and could now not even negotiate the three steps from her hospital bed to a toilet without the assistance of myself and two hospital attendants. The nurses, as seems to always be the case, were fabulous. In fact, one of the nurses addressed us in a personal fashion when the doctor had left the room. She told us to not be worried by his attitude; she would take care of us. I cannot underestimate the importance of a friendly face when faced with medical catastrophes. No one wants to come to an emergency room, we come only when necessary. And although I would dearly love to have the "private" insurance this particular doctor craved, I could not forget the fact of Debbie's "private" insurance dropping her as soon as she was diagnosed and placing us in the position we were now in. I am thankful for governmental programs such as Medicare and Medicaid. They have kept Debbie alive when the private insurance companies would have denied her treatment because she was no longer profitable to them.

The doctor was mandated by policy to hold Debbie for observation and we spent 12 hours in the emergency room but the doctor would not admit her and he insisted upon our leaving the premises when the 12 hours had expired. He never offered any explanation for the change in Debbie's demeanor nor did he offer any suggestions as to how we should proceed further. Fortunately, I had insisted that a copy of the CAT scan be forwarded to Duke.

It turns out Debbie suffered a mild concussion when she banged her head against the back wall of the shower stall. It took nearly three months for Debbie to regain the ability of unassisted walking. We returned to Virginia's following the hospital visit. Debbie's concussion led to my losing much sleep in the immediate days that came next and I lost whatever composure I still had left.

A week or so following her fall in the shower I was a sincerely ragged individual. I was angry and try as I might that anger spilled from my mouth almost every time I opened it. I was baffled by Debbie's inability to move herself and for the first time began to consider seriously that I was incompetent to care for Debbie. I did not have the skills and it was apparent that I no longer had the stamina and patience that I would need. I felt horrible. I wondered if I would be able to keep Debbie from a nursing home for much longer.

Before our travel to Florida I had discussed with Virginia that sometime during our stay I would like to leave Debbie in her care for a few days while I went camping in a nearby state park. Virginia was completely fine with that but Debbie's fall had changed the situation radically. Debbie now needed active support each time she attempted to waddle through the house.

Now, I love my mother-in-law. Virginia is a remarkable woman. At eighty-eight years young she still lived alone in her own house, did her own cooking, cleaning and shopping. She still drives her own vehicle. It terrifies me to ride along with her, as she seemingly believes that her current age is also the legal speed limit. She will hit 88 miles per hour between the stop signs in her neighborhood. I swear that when I first met her sixteen years ago she only drove at 72 miles per hour! Fortunately, Florida streets are long and straight. Virginia worked as a nurse her entire life, switching to home care nursing when she was in her seventies. She worked full time until her 85th year. If anyone should have known the limitations of a brain cancer patient, it is she. The problem was that she just could not accept that it was her daughter who needed such help.

It is a very thin line between allowing a patient (Debbie!) the independence to maintain as normal a lifestyle as possible and in creating and enforcing policies that will ensure her safety. I have walked that line now for ten years and I tend to lean toward safety and risk management in my effort to keep Debbie happy and unhurt. Virginia, although loving and well meaning, had not been witness to all of the preventable falls that I had seen. In the case of Debbie's shower, we were in complete disagreement.

One evening Virginia sensed my frustration and suggested that I leave the following morning on the camping trip I had planned. I asked her, "Who will take care of Debbie?"

"I will", she responded.

"What will you do when she falls?" This was not a silly question. Virginia could see Debbie's needing a strong arm to support her during the day. She did not see the struggle I had every two hours each night to get Debbie safely to the commode. Debbie was, and still is, most vulnerable when she first awakes and has not yet gotten her body to respond to her mind's commands. Even with all the love in the world Virginia was not able to support Debbie's weight with her frail and aged body.

"I'll get help, I'll call my neighbor."

"And you'll do that several times a night while Debbie waits and needs to pee?" I was incredulous. I knew Virginia could not do what she so hoped she would be able to and I couldn't make her see that. I didn't mean to, and I certainly regretted my action almost instantly, but the dam burst and I erupted in a loud and angry torrent of abuse at a sweet, old woman who had shown me nothing but kindness.

"God damn it, if you had just supported me and not encouraged Debbie to shower alone she wouldn't have fallen in the first place!" I went on for several minutes, loudly and out of control. There was usage of several words that should never have been spoken. I was right, of course, but even righteous anger must be tempered with kindness and compassion and I had none left. Thankfully I did not hit or break anyone or anything. Virginia asked me to leave and cool off. I did, driving fast and furiously for nearly a hundred miles before the lateness of the hour forced me to stop at a rest area and nap for an hour. I was back in the house by three in the morning. My first chore was to take Debbie to the commode and change the sheets on Debbie's wet bed.

Debbie celebrated her birthday two weeks after the fall. I had arranged with her sisters, Jennifer and Robin, to have a surprise party for Debbie at Jennifer's home in Sarasota. I had contacted Debbie's nieces and nephews and was thrilled when Brooke and Amber said that they could join us from Jacksonville along with the rest of Debbie's extended family who lived nearby to Virginia. I was glad that Debbie's family had gathered on her behalf. They do not get together often enough.

Of course, the word of my tantrum had gotten around and I was a pariah and an outsider at a party and family reunion that I had organized myself. In illustration of this I offer this tidbit. I had set our arrival at Jennifer's in the late afternoon to allow time for those who were traveling to arrive before us so that Debbie's surprise would be complete. Virginia decided arbitrarily to call Debbie's sisters and their children to come in the early afternoon. She did not believe me when I told her that Brooke and Amber were coming from Jacksonville. Like I said, Debbie's family does not gather often. Anyway, I was able to contact our nieces and got them to hasten their departure and I held Debbie back until I had been informed of everyone's arrival. This required some fancy storytelling to Debbie as the logistics for the day changed almost every hour.

The surprise for Debbie was delightful and the evening was a joyous one for Debbie. I had convinced Debbie that the reason we were driving to her sister's was because Jennifer had agreed to join us for a birthday dinner. Debbie received the love and honor from her family that she so rightfully deserves. Although distressed by the apparent weakness that Debbie exhibited her family showered her with affection. I was glad to step back and let her relatives assist her as the evening progressed.

Virginia and I did reconcile before Debbie and I left for home. I am sorry I had such a blow up but Virginia did come to recognize the effort I was constantly exerting on Debbie's behalf and she did acknowledge that she was unable physically to provide as I was. We continue to speak to one another frequently by telephone and I sincerely hope that our visit this year will not have the fireworks and explosions.

For the next three months, in Florida and also after a difficult ride home, Debbie did not once go to the rest room without my supporting her weight on my increasingly painful back. Until nearly the beginning of June we were unable to go anywhere or do anything. Somehow and thankfully Debbie's will overcame her infirmity and she learned once more to do something we all take for granted- to take a step.

CHAPTER 4

The first thing we did upon arriving home was to obtain a shower transfer seat. This is a chair that sits in the tub and has a bench that extends from the tub so that Debbie can sit on the bench and slide herself into the shower. She still needs help getting in and out from the shower, but at least she can safely scrub herself without my constant presence. This is a great relief to us both and we are thankful to our local Senior Citizen's Center for making this piece of equipment available to us at a nominal fee.

We also restarted Debbie's program of physical therapy. This once again became incredibly important. Debbie's concussion had caused another severe jar to her equilibrium and much work was needed for her to regain her balance. We returned to a program of exercise and it is a blessing that through effort and hard work Debbie has once again become able to walk in our local park and on other flat, wide trails. It takes Debbie nearly three times as long to walk a half-mile loop. I thought we were slow when that distance took us nearly 40 minutes. Now it takes anywhere between 90 minutes and two hours depending on how long Debbie chooses to remain at each of the benches we sit on as we make our revolution.

I must acknowledge the kindness of Debbie's brother Brad who has been willing to sacrifice an occasional weekend to care for Debbie and allow me to getaway. His help in April permitted me to attend the Merlefest bluegrass festival where for three days I almost felt as if I had not a care in the world. I am sure that the respite does help rejuvenate me but I must admit that the reality of my return home to a weakened Debbie is a depressing and shattering blow. Within minutes I am back on full responsibility mode and the glow of my time away dissolves immediately.

Our summer has been amazingly calm. Once Debbie relearned how to walk we once more tried to utilize our location to great advantage. My choice, long ago, to live in the Blue Ridge has served me well and Debbie's insistence upon our marriage to join me here has allowed us to live in what I truly feel is the most beautiful part of our country. Yet I mourn the loss of the carefree attitude I had when I was younger. Sometimes the realities of the things I have lost overpower me and I do not respond well.

One hot evening in August, only a few weeks from our 15th wedding anniversary and the 10th anniversary of Debbie's cancer, she was working quietly beading another of the necklaces that she loves to create. I slipped away to the bathroom and heard the unmistakable boom of Debbie collapsing to the floor. I hastily zipped up my shorts and came running to help her. She was unhurt. This was your typical garden-variety fall; Debbie had not hit her head and she asked me to help her back up and into her chair. After I did so I asked her how she had happened to fall this time. This is a process we go through each time to help Debbie recognize patterns in order to prevent her falls. She told me she had dropped a bead that had rolled into the corner by the television set.

For what must be by now the five thousandth time I reminded Debbie of the safety rule I had created. "Stay out of corners!" I reminded her again that I am always just seconds away and that all she had to do was be patient enough to allow me to finish in the bathroom and that she could then ask for my help. I reminded her, once again, that I would much prefer to help her with a small thing than to be forced to help her by lifting her off the ground. Debbie reiterated that she had gone in search of a lost bead. Once more I asked her to consider the consequence and potential danger of her actions. She insisted the bead was more important than my safety rule. Debbie had already forgotten that she would be on the floor still if I hadn't helped her up. The only thing she could focus on was the wandering bead that was still lying underneath the television stand. She demanded that I retrieve it for her immediately.

"Fuck the bead and fuck you!" Debbie's complete disregard for her own safety and her firmness in her own righteousness had lit my fuse. For the next ten minutes or so I was ballistic. I was shouting at the top of my lungs using obscenities strung together in compound fashion. I had no idea of what I was saying; I was just a volcano exploding in a vile spew of ugliness. I know that Debbie has no fear of my ever striking her. I am totally incapable of ever doing so but this venting of venom did finally pierce her. She began to cry. She apologized for disregarding my rule for her safety. We hugged and Debbie kissed my cheek and then padded off to bed. I sat in the kitchen by the computer screen trying to catch my breath, wipe away my tears and lose myself in a computer game.

An hour later there was a knock on the front screen door of our house. It was an officer from the county sheriff's office. One of our neighbors had heard my tirade through the open windows on this sultry summer's eve. The indiscriminate language I had been using offended our neighbors and they called the police. The next hour will forever remain the most embarrassing hour of my entire life.

There is a television program called Cops during which actual footage of patrolmen at work is shown. My driveway resembled a Cops episode on this particular night. I answered the knock wearing nothing but a pair of cut off shorts. I was shocked to see the sheriff standing on my porch. He informed me that he was responding to a call involving a domestic dispute and asked if I could tell him what had happened. I could see his vehicle parked halfway down the drive and could sense that the entire hillside was watching and listening to the drama now taking place in my yard and where I was the main culprit.

Immediately I began to explain what had happened. "My wife is a brain cancer patient and I was angry with her because she disobeyed a safety directive and could have been seriously hurt."

The officer interrupted and said, "You must be under a lot of stress."

I chuckled at his understatement and told him that he didn't have half a clue as to the amount of emotional stress I live with constantly. He assured me that he was there to help us and asked if he could step inside to talk with Debbie.

I told him that Debbie had already gone to bed but that I would wake her and bring her to him. I asked him if he would mind waiting on the porch and offered him a glass of water or soda. The officer explained that a second sheriff was on his way and that upon his arrival they would speak with Debbie and I separately. He asked if that would be OK with me and I agreed that would be fine. The next twenty minutes found me returning to and from the officer on my front porch and Debbie's bedroom. I gave him a running commentary on the progression of Debbie's arising, using the bathroom, and getting dressed. I made sure I spoke clearly enough so that he could hear me telling Debbie who was visiting. Debbie was tickled when she finally came out and saw the two sheriff's deputies awaiting her arrival. She smiled at the two men and bent over to read their nametags, and then called them by name and said "Good evening" to each of them. I just cracked up laughing. I couldn't help doing that either. Debbie's childlike greeting just released all the pressure and my tenseness dissipated.

The next thirty minutes my officer and I spoke of possible programs that I could look into to help with my issues of being a 24/7 caregiver. The officer was trying his best to be helpful but it was excruciating for us both. Each program he mentioned was one I was already familiar with. He went down his list and I explained how each program was no longer able to fulfill its goals due to recent budget costs. I mentioned names of people I had spoken with and he recognized I was telling the truth. We do live in a small community and eventually you know everyone. And that was the worst of the whole ordeal. I do not recommend meeting police officers for the first time when they are responding to a call at which you are the only possible offender. A few years earlier I might have met those same two officers at a school outing. I was thoroughly ashamed and apologized for taking up their valuable time.

Apparently the officer who interviewed Debbie was satisfied with her responses as he came down the drive and said that everything was fine. They wished us luck and invited us to call them should we ever require their assistance. Debbie did relay to me later that the only question the officer asked her was- "Did he hit you?" Her response was, "Of course not!"

It's been over three months since then. It was a month before I could even begin to see any humor in that situation at all. Now Debbie and I are able to laugh about it and now when she blatantly violates a safety rule I just say, "OK, Debbie, might as well just pick up the phone and call your buddies, Officers B. and H., because I am really pissed off at you."

Of course nobody lives in a bubble. Debbie and I are surrounded by neighbors and by our countrymen and this year has not been the best of times for people like us who have worked our lives paying into programs like Social Security, Medicare and health insurance. Many folks feel we are to blame for the bad economic times we are living through. I do not accept that. There has been much talk of 99% vs. 1%. Let there be no doubt, Debbie and I are solidly with the 99%.

More so than most we have witnessed the results of corporations being coddled and allowed to do as they see fit. The only thing a corporation sees fit to do is to make profit. This is right and proper. But is it right and proper for insurance companies to drop a client when that client must make a claim? Shouldn't they be forced to pay the bills when legitimate claims are presented? People's health should not be dependent on the whims of corporate interest. Taking the profit motive out of the health care system will benefit us all. People before profits, peace before war. I still believe, as I did a year ago, that the soul of the American people is a kind one. We do care about each other, now we need to find a way to join together and ensure that our private values of love and compassion find their way back into the fabric of our society. We have nothing to fear from government as long as we all remember that the government is nothing more than us.

The most amazing thing to happen to us this year is that I have written a book and that you are reading it! I sincerely never knew I had it in me to complete such a project. If I had been assigned to write this, I don't believe it would ever have seen the light of day. I have been flattered by the responses of those readers who have chosen to contact me. I hope to be able to maintain friendships with all of you. You are incredible and I am thrilled that our story has touched you. I never dreamed that Debbie would have the opportunity to hear her story read aloud and that she would be able to witness firsthand the responses to her courage from total strangers. Thank you for joining us on our journey. I wish you happiness, joy and health. I apologize for my imperfections and hope you never have to suffer from the guilt and depression I struggle with constantly.

Have I failed? Perhaps not. I still waken each day with hope and expectation of joy for both Debbie and myself. I continue to do my best and pray that it is enough.

ABOUT THE AUTHOR

The author was born in Brooklyn, N.Y. where he played sports in the street as a child while dodging moving vehicles. He met and married his first wife after meeting her at summer camp. He traveled with his wife to a North Carolina mountain town where his wife took a graduate degree, slept around a bit and then returned to the big city. The author remained in the Blue Ridge, met and courted his second wife Debbie and worked at various and sundry jobs. He still resides in the Blue Ridge to this day. He enjoys most music, walking through the outdoors, baseball, the pristine quiet of a snowy day in the mountains and a cold beer on hot summer afternoons.
The author can be reached at:

tinroofinn@yahoo.com

He looks forward to hearing from you and responding to your correspondence. He thanks you for reading and encourages you to write.

www.ingramcontent.com/pod-product-compliance
Lightning Source LLC
Chambersburg PA
CBHW081130170526

45165CB00008B/2623

* 9 7 8 1 4 6 3 7 7 9 3 9 9 *